PRAISE

MIDPOINT:

MANHOOD, MIDLIFE, AND PROSTATE CANCER

"Hill's *Midpoint* is a poignant account of a man's journey with prostate cancer and an insightful glimpse into the complexity of men's health. His rawness and vulnerability make his memoir both engaging and relatable. *Midpoint* is a courageous work, valuable to all men with prostate cancer and to the people who love them."

—ELAINE HOLT, MD, author of *The Doctor Next Door*

"Jim Hill has written a wonderfully honest journey to follow for anyone who has or is dealing with not only prostate cancer but any form of cancer."

—JULIE MACNEIL, award-winning author of *The 50-Year Secret*

"James Hill's engaging memoir, *Midpoint Manhood, Midlife and Prostate Cancer*, is his very personal story of how a prostate cancer diagnosis influenced his relationships and his own views of himself and of masculinity. He shares his fears, his setbacks, and his successes that are common to many of us who have traveled this same path. Having Jim's first-hand account will prove invaluable to the newly diagnosed prostate cancer patient and is relevant to those who have been dealing with this disease for some time."

—DAN ZELLER, author of *Dan's Journey through Prostate Cancer* (blog), www.dansjourney.com

Midpoint:
Manhood, Midlife, and Prostate Cancer

by James A. Hill

© Copyright 2019 James A. Hill

ISBN 978-1-63393-833-5

Published by

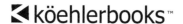

210 60th Street
Virginia Beach, VA 23451
800—435—4811
www.koehlerbooks.com

MIDPOINT

MANHOOD
MIDLIFE
AND
PROSTATE
CANCER

JAMES A. HILL

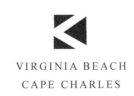

VIRGINIA BEACH
CAPE CHARLES

To the nearly 165,000 American men who will be diagnosed with prostate cancer this year. If even one of them finds this book remotely useful or encouraging, it will have done its job.

To protect their privacy, I have used pseudonyms for a number of individuals referred to in this book.

INTRODUCTION

I WAS SITTING ALONE in Examination Room 3, naked from the waist down, with a white sheet on my lap to cover my groin and upper thighs. My private parts, which were the subject of this appointment, had already begun a tactical retreat, as male genitalia tend to do in cold swimming pools and under fluorescent lights. Waiting for the door to open, I sat there like a kid in the principal's office, my legs dangling twelve inches off the floor. At one point, it occurred to me that my navy blue socks were pulled up over my calves, which must have looked ridiculous; so I hopped off the seat and pushed them down so they bunched casually around my ankles. Rearranging deck chairs on the Titanic, I mused. This is what things had come to.

My appointment that day was at the Sexual Health clinic of Memorial Sloan Kettering Cancer Center in New York City. Roughly three months before that, I had been diagnosed with stage-3 prostate cancer. A month after my diagnosis, I had a nerve-sparing laparoscopic radical prostatectomy at MSK's Memorial Hospital a few blocks away. Now, after a rather long and unexpectedly complicated odyssey, I was about to meet with Naomi, one of the nurse practitioners on MSK's Sexual Health team. To be clear, "sexual health" in the context of prostate cancer is all about the quality of one's erections. After you've had your prostate removed, your hard-ons become a subject of considerable scrutiny. That's because the delicate process of removing a prostate—the walnut-sized gland tucked right down in the middle of everything that matters to a man—can leave a guy impotent and incontinent for weeks, months, or even permanently. So here I was to ensure that any "challenges" I faced as a result of my surgery would be measured in months, not years.

Before being shown into Examination Room 3, I filled out a long questionnaire about everything related to my sexual activity. In another life, I couldn't have imagined answering those questions for anyone. But here I was, eight weeks after having my cancer-ridden walnut removed, and I had become an open book. I answered every question with cheerful resignation. They asked about the quality and frequency of erections. Did I attempt intercourse? How did it go? Did I masturbate? Did I have orgasms? Were they satisfying? How was my self-esteem? Had I lost any length in my penis? All kinds of humiliating stuff. Way beyond trying to bluff on anything, I answered as honestly as I could. Besides, in a moment Naomi would come in and we would talk about all of this in person, with nothing more than a cotton sheet between her questions and the stark light of truth.

As I waited for Naomi, I glanced under the sheet to see how things would look when the big reveal occurred. The room was reasonably warm, which any man would appreciate in such a situation. Plus I didn't have a catheter in (more on that later), which makes your johnson look oddly bionic, like something under the hood of a Toyota. As the irony gods would have it, Naomi was both young and attractive and, to make matters worse, she was pregnant—I'm guessing six or seven months along. So not only did she represent youth and beauty—both of which seemed to have vanished from my own identity—but she was the very picture of sexual and reproductive vitality.

Naomi was very pleasant, as the staff at MSK tended to be. She apologized for the wait and asked me to review how things had gone since my surgery. I walked her through the major developments, keeping it businesslike but friendly. Then she launched into more questions about my "sexual health," getting even more granular than the questionnaire had been, if that were possible. Again, I answered with as much candor as I could muster, cracking very few awkward jokes, though the temptation was overwhelming at times. I hadn't talked this much about my private parts since I was in a fraternity, and never with such deadly seriousness. Naomi listened intently, taking notes as I went. So far, she didn't seem interested in removing the sheet, which was a relief. Even when she began the physical examination, her focus was on my blood pressure and listening to my heart and lungs under my sweater. She took a few more notes and sat back down on the stool in front of me.

"Okay, let's take a quick look . . . " she said, breezily drawing back the sheet.

By that point, I was accustomed to dropping my trousers for pretty much anyone in a white coat and blue rubber gloves. But it never failed to amaze me how poker-faced these professionals could be in such an otherwise absurd encounter. Here I was, a complete stranger Naomi might have bumped into on the elevator not fifteen minutes earlier and who, in an act of middle-aged gallantry, might have asked her, "What floor?" As the elevator dinged at the fourth floor, she might have smiled at him and said "Thanks" as he stepped aside to let her exit first. In this moment of gender-normative convention, both parties play a comfortable and coherent role that safeguards the privacy and dignity of each. Notably, both parties are fully clothed.

How these dynamics change when one of those individuals is naked from the waist down. Remove the man's pants and he is no longer a courteous man on the elevator but has become a vulnerable, slightly ridiculous figure in rumpled socks.

Naomi, I assumed, must look at men's genitals all day long. She probably overcame her initial hesitation to remove the fateful sheet—that tense moment of exposing an adult male to her professional scrutiny—back during her medical training. But for every man who comes into her examining room for the first time, it's a moment of peculiar unease that harkens a new, unglamorous phase of life. No longer is your manhood viewed with tenderness in the dim light of a bedroom. There was no pride in this unveiling. Since my diagnosis, disrobing in the presence of others had become an antiseptic matter in which I was the object not of desire but of clinical scrutiny and a touch of compassion. It turns out, centuries of exalting the male phallus in Roman and Greek statuary come to naught in Examination Room 3. Here, for all the attempts by caregivers to treat me like a healing human being (and at MSK they worked hard to do that), I felt more like a troubled length of garden hose in need of repair.

The next phase of the examination went quickly. With her years of experience, Naomi must have understood how uncomfortable men are in such a situation. She worked efficiently with blue-gloved hands, conducting various stretches and palpitations. Then, to my relief, she replaced the sheet. Things had gone well to that point and I figured I'd be safely back in trousers in no time.

"So the tissue looks pretty healthy down there and our timing is good, starting so soon after surgery."

Starting? I thought to myself.

"I'm going to recommend we begin penile injections . . . " I'm pretty sure she said a lot more after "penile injections," but all I heard was the furious rush of blood pounding in my ears.

"I realize," Naomi was saying, somewhere at the end of a tunnel, "that injections don't sound great at first, but most men report tolerating them very well and getting excellent results."

"For how long?"

"Two to three times per week for a year."

It's amazing how quickly you can do math when it involves sticking a needle in your penis. That was 156 discrete puncture wounds in my sacred man-self. How, I wondered, could inflicting that kind of damage actually help matters?

As I regained my composure, Naomi explained that during prostate surgery, the doctor's objective is to remove *all* the cancer, even if doing so results in collateral damage to nearby tissue and nerves. In my case, the surgeon, Dr. Touijer, performed a "nerve-sparing radical prostatectomy," in which he removed the prostate, nearby lymph nodes, seminal vesicles, and tissue around the prostate where the cancer had encroached— all while avoiding the nerves required for achieving an erection. However, even under the best circumstances, the surgeon must peel the nerve bundles off the prostate, stretch and maneuver them, clamp them, and set them aside while he removes the gland. Then he un-clamps the nerves and relocates them to rest along the "pelvic bed." All this inflicts considerable trauma. My cancer had come very close to the left nerve bundle, so there had been some additional, though limited, damage there. She went on to explain that, even when the nerve bundles in your groin aren't affected, all that jostling about causes nerves to go into "hibernation mode" for one or two *years*. During that time, they simply don't want to participate in whatever sexual inclinations you have. The result can be prolonged periods without an erection. And because the penis is like a muscle, the old adage of "use it or lose it" applies rather ominously—both to one's ability to achieve an erection and to maintain one's overall length. Both these concepts, most men will agree, are near and dear to male confidence. Simply put, penile tissue needs to be utilized regularly—stretched and filled with fresh, oxygenated blood—or that tissue atrophies. Permanently.

She now had my undivided attention. Naomi explained that penile injections dilate the arteries in the penis and allow blood to flow in and "mechanically" create an erection, which stretches the tissue and keeps it healthy while the nerves recover. When the healing process is complete, the injections are discontinued and life goes on, theoretically, with minimal assistance from needles or pills. At least, that's the goal. Naomi answered all my questions—and there were many. We agreed I'd come back to New York City later that week for back-to-back appointments to begin my "rehabilitation." I was comforted by her use of that term. It helped me see myself not as damaged but as coming back from an injury—like a running back rehabbing a torn ACL. It was a reach, but it helped.

When I returned to the Sexual Health practice that following Thursday, I was trying to focus on this concept of "rehab." This, I reminded myself, was all about returning to my previous robust physical and sexual health. If it meant some discomfort and loss of privacy (and dignity) for a while, I could man up. It would be worth it. That was my mindset when Rob walked into the examination room to give me my first shot. I liked him immediately. He was about my age, maybe a little younger, balding with white cropped hair and stylish glasses. He was casually but fashionably dressed under his white coat. I remember noticing his topsiders and colorful socks as he spoke to me. He was reassuring without being saccharine. Something in his demeanor made me speculate he was gay, which I found calming—maybe because I associated gay men with an absence of heterosexual bravado. That suited me just fine at the moment.

"I know," Rob began, "that 'needle' and 'penis' don't go well in a sentence together."

You got that right, I thought.

"But I've trained thousands of men on injections, and on a scale of 1 to 10 for pain, on average they report feeling a 1.5 to 2. Really. Most men almost don't feel anything." Sloan Kettering uses this 1-to-10 scale on lots of things, it turns out, including the intensity of pain and, as I would come to learn, the quality of one's erections.

As he spoke, Rob prepared the syringe with practiced efficiency, explaining everything he was doing and reassuring me at every step. Mostly he used clinical language when talking about my anatomy, but every now and then, he'd say, "hard on" or "dick," to remind me that he, too, was a guy with a penis. On some level he had to empathize with my predicament. Long story short, the shot turned out to be a solid 8 on the pain scale, but the "bee sting" on the left side of my penis quickly faded. I may have startled some people in the waiting room when I screamed "Sweet Jesus," but after that I was pretty composed. To be fair to Rob, the alarming pain I felt was from an excess of alcohol on the injection site, and his claim that the injections aren't terribly painful was, mercifully, true. The shot administered, it was just a matter of letting the medication work its magic and gauging the results. So, I sat on the exam room chair with the sheet in my lap with Rob popping in every fifteen minutes or so to see how things were "coming along."

As things came along, Rob conducted a turgidity assessment, bending the flagpole in question to gauge where it stood on the 1-to-10 "quality" scale. Before he gave me his verdict, he asked my opinion.

"I don't know . . . six or seven?"

"No, that's an eight."

Despite my best poker face, I may have smiled a little.

As Rob completed his evaluation, it occurred to me I had experienced another first in this cancer saga, which in any other context would have been nothing short of a game-changer: Another man had just complimented me on how stiff my erection was.

Definitely new territory.

It has been a long, strange trip, indeed. As I entered the whirlwind that occasions a scary medical diagnosis, I couldn't help but feel that, as a culture, we're not entirely honest with ourselves about how prostate cancer treatment goes. Much about my treatment was consistent with what I read in the disastrously written book my urologist gave me, or the websites and blogs I haunted. And yet so much was completely unexpected. In all the reading I did to prepare for that journey—and I did a lot—I kept feeling that so much about prostate cancer gets glossed over, euphemized, or simplified. We talk of prostate cancer as the "good cancer" and, in doing so, fail to candidly address the not-so-good complications that come with its treatment. The popular press tells us that prostate cancer survival rates are high because it's an indolent malignancy that goes about its business as aimlessly as a man doing Saturday chores while watching The Masters on television. Optimism about prostate treatment has become so commonplace in our collective mythology that we think of men cheerfully heading off to have the problematic gland removed or irradiated, returning for a couple days of rest on the couch, and *voila!*, back to the desk job at Allstate.

Further coloring our cultural view of prostate cancer—and in a troubling way—is its association with old age. We hear statistics, many of which feel like urban legend by now, that many elderly men have undiagnosed prostate cancer when they die. One study published in 2015 looked at the prevalence of undiagnosed prostate cancer at autopsy, noting that, among men aged 70-79, tumor was found in 36 percent of Caucasians and 51 percent of African-Americans. From these data points, we might conclude that for many men the best strategy is "watchful waiting," where one forgoes treatment in favor of monitoring. After all, if you're already old, you'll probably die of something else before the cancer does any harm. We hear stories of incontinence and impotence, of old men wearing diapers under their khakis to avoid untimely leaking on the living room couch. As a middle-aged man, I had heard those stories and unfairly made the mental connection between prostate cancer and elderly male bodies that were already falling apart: Their plumbing didn't work anymore as it was, so what was the big deal about an absorbent pad in the Jockeys? As for post-surgical erectile dysfunction, how often does a 75-year-old man need a hard-on? The fact that prostate cancer affects older men has somehow resulted in its being viewed through layers of bias and euphemism. Perhaps those layers are the result of multitudes of stoical men who don't want their vulnerability on display. Perhaps women in our male-dominated culture, who are beset by their own panoply of horrific cancers, have been too willing to accept those euphemisms unquestioningly. And perhaps there's a healthy dose of ageism informing all of this, as well.

As if these considerations aren't enough to complicate the subject of prostate cancer, a significant new factor emerged the year I was diagnosed—one that colored how I viewed my disease and how American culture, in turn, viewed me. On October 15, 2017, ten days after *The New York Times* published an article on Harvey Weinstein's alleged decades of sexual misconduct—and about two months before I was diagnosed—actress Alyssa Milano took to Twitter to encourage her followers to use the term "me too" to share their experiences of sexual assault and harassment. By the next day, #metoo had been tweeted more than 500,000 times. Facebook blew up as well, with twelve million posts containing the hashtag appearing in the first twenty-four hours after Milano's tweet. Over the course of the next few months, dozens of high-profile men in politics, entertainment, and business were toppled from power as accusations of their sexual misconduct emerged. Justifiable anger exploded around the globe against male hegemony and unaccountability. In the midst of this cultural maelstrom, I received one alarming test result after another, leaving me feeling sexually humbled and far from powerful—a vulnerability that contradicted the prevailing narrative in the world around me. My uniquely male medical concern in the age of #metoo was both invisible and inconsequential. When I was inclined to talk more broadly about prostate cancer and middle age, I drew back. If males really were such brutes, one might have concluded, perhaps it was fitting that the number-two cancer killer of men can rob us of our sexual potency and urinary continence. That kind of thinking was, of course, paranoid and unfairly gender-abnegating. Still, in the angry zeitgeist of late 2017 and early 2018, it was hard to imagine anyone wanting to hear me, or any man, complain about prostate cancer.

Euphemism, ageism—and now anger—contribute to a collective cultural misrepresentation, or even non-representation, of prostate cancer and treatment. And we are all, to some extent, complicit. Sociologists would surely argue that these dynamics find their origins in "gender construction" and how American men and women are socialized from birth to perform rigid gender roles and reject gender "displays" that contradict those roles. Men are programmed to be providers, leaders, and aggressors. Reduced to gender stereotypes, however, we can be seen as taciturn, animalistic, and sexually brutish. While men will talk endlessly about tearing a meniscus playing touch football, they clam up when it comes to more sensitive health issues, particularly those that make them feel vulnerable. In that sense, we men are unwitting culprits in promulgating our own worst stereotypes. But nobody benefits from viewing 50 percent of humanity as mechanical beings who eat, defecate, get hard, ejaculate, and fall asleep. Meanwhile, the same culture that totalizes male sexuality invests women's bodies with a kind of mystical spirituality conferred by the awe-inspiring ability to create and carry life. I believe women's bodies are absolutely amazing. I remember witnessing the birth of my daughter, Madeleine, after something like 24 hours of labor. Afterward, I told my exhausted wife she seemed like an Olympic athlete and that her stamina and toughness humbled me. I bought into the whole idea that women's bodies are astonishingly complex, life-giving, and nuanced organisms. And yet, don't men participate in the miracle of reproduction as well? Don't male bodies have a touch of the divine, some of the same unfathomable complexity? Until I was diagnosed with a disease of the male reproductive system, it never occurred to me that my own body might be nuanced, even delicate, in its own way.

My mother died of breast cancer when she was only 42. After a grueling mastectomy and six years in remission, the cancer returned with a ferocity, claiming her in 1969. Breast cancer is a horrific, dehumanizing disease that robs women of a fundamental part of their feminine identity. We read about the devastating impact a mastectomy has on a woman's sense of self—on her identity as a woman, her sexuality, her entire being. The healing process for a woman is every bit as psychological as it is physical. No wonder: The breast, with its ability to give life-sustaining nourishment to a child, is perhaps the most enduring emblem of womanhood. For the man, that emblem is his penis—not as we see it on Michelangelo's David where it is more incidental to the overall picture of pulchritude, but as the erect phallus, gorged with life-giving power. The phallus has been fetishized over the centuries for its fundamental representation of male viability; and the masculine ego has, both historically and biologically, revolved around it. Take that emblem of male pride away from a man and, make no mistake, he is traumatized. Gender roles, however, make it unlikely he will talk about this trauma, even with his closest friends. It's just too revealing. Therein lies at least one cause for our collective glossing-over of male angst in the age of prostate cancer.

When preparing for this book, I did some casual research on the representation of the penis in classical statuary and came across an anecdote that perfectly emblematized cultural attitudes toward male sexuality. In 1857, the Grand Duke of Tuscany, in an act of diplomatic goodwill toward England, had a full-size plaster cast of Michelangelo's David produced and delivered to the fledgling South Kensington Museum (which later became the Victoria and Albert Museum) in London. The story goes that when Queen Victoria first viewed this remarkable gift, she was shocked by David's state of unapologetic nudity. Consequently, the museum commissioned a proportionate half-meter-long plaster fig leaf which, by means of strategically located hooks, was hung over David's private parts whenever royalty visited. Though we've come a long way since Victoria first blushed at David's penis, we've got more progress to make before male sexuality is discussed with the candor and subtlety it deserves. The surprisingly nuanced reality of manhood, like the genitals under the fig leaf, becomes no less real or nuanced just because we drape it in euphemism, obscure it in stereotypes, or dismiss it out of contempt.

On a recent train ride back from an appointment at Sloan Kettering, I was browsing the news feed on my iPhone. I came across a *New York Times* article tantalizingly entitled, "What Sleeping With Married Men Taught Me About Infidelity," by Karin Jones. The article wasn't really my cup of tea, but I read it because it made some interesting points about men, their sexual and emotional needs, and how they sometimes resort to infidelity rather than have candid discussions with their wives about each other's sexual needs. Then I came across a line that, sadly, summarizes the view our culture so often takes of male sexuality:

> *We all go through phases of wanting it and not wanting it. I doubt most women avoid having sex with their husbands because they lack physical desire in general; we are simply more complex sexual animals. Which is why men can get an erection from a pill but there's no way to medically induce arousal and desire in women.*

To hear Karin Jones tell it, men are simply more basic "sexual animals." Give us a little blue pill, point us in the right direction, and, *presto*, we're ready to rock 'n' roll. But does an artificially functioning erection really correct the constellation of emotional and physical problems associated with sexual dysfunction? Male sexuality, it turns out, is complicated too. Just the act of achieving an erection is a minor miracle of physiology. As my surgeon explained to me, an erection requires three physical components: blood flow, functioning nerves, and proper hormone levels. But even with those three factors working in a carefully balanced harmony (which is more and more difficult for the aging body to achieve), all you get is a stiff dick. The physiological erection speaks only to part of the male sexual experience. There remains the complicated matter of his emotional involvement and his reaction, or lack thereof, to and interaction with sources of arousal, whether they be visual, physical, or psychological. Stimuli and physiology all need to work in concert to prepare for and consummate the sex act and, ultimately, to actualize the male sexual identity. Remove one of those critical components, and the symphony of sexual potency is silenced.

If a pill can resurrect the wounded phallus, what repairs the damage to a man's self-esteem? His sense of his virility? What about the loss of spontaneity, or the reliance on medication to achieve a marginal erection? If a woman is devastated by the loss of her breast, is a man any less devastated by the loss, whether temporary or permanent, of *his* emblem of sexual vitality, the proud erection?

On top of all this, a man without a prostate has what the medical profession refers to as "anejaculation," which means that when he has an orgasm, nothing comes out of his penis. The prostate is central to the production of semen and without it, well, you get the idea. It's like penile dry heaves. And without the feeling of "fullness" that comes with semen building up in the urethra prior to ejaculation, orgasms become, for most men, much less intense. Gone, too, is the visual satisfaction of *seeing* an explosive ejaculation.

In addition to sexual dysfunction or diminution, there is the matter of post-prostatectomy incontinence. Whether it's the occasional occurrence of "stress incontinence"—an errant drip when you sneeze or stand up suddenly—or constant leakage requiring surgical intervention, any loss of urinary control is devastating to male confidence. The same problem that causes incontinence also contributes, for some men, to a strange new phenomenon during sex. My nurse practitioner Naomi disclosed that it's not uncommon for men who undergo prostate surgery to squirt urine from their penises when they have an orgasm. Now *there's* a detail you don't read about on sunny prostate cancer websites. So abundant are these "issues" that many cancer patients I met based their treatment decisions primarily on the odds of avoiding one side effect or another. After all, I've heard men say, "What's the point of lengthening your life if you have to wear diapers or can't get it up anymore?"

All this is to say that the subject of prostate cancer is a good deal more complicated than I realized when I first got the phone call that my PSA was high. And as I've learned just *how* complicated, and how so little candor exists in conversations about prostate cancer, I decided to share some of my own experience. Certain things I experienced have been, as I said, pretty textbook. Many of my emotional responses were anticipated in literature I read. But much of what I experienced were big surprises to me. What's more, my cancer hit me at a midpoint in life when, for many men, you're starting to feel a creeping sense of obsolescence, whether in your career, your athletic pursuits, even your appearance. It's a time when men are already having to modify personal narratives previously built on rising trajectories; they must come to terms with diminished professional prestige, declining earning power, fading sexual potency, aching joints, sore muscles, gray or thinning hair, tenacious belly fat, and a general sense that life just isn't what it used to be. In other words, it can be a pretty physically and psychologically challenging time on its own. A prostate cancer diagnosis can underscore all those dark dynamics in a way that makes life particularly unappealing—and unexpectedly fraught.

Calling prostate cancer "the good cancer" is a cheerful way for the medical profession to encourage men not to freak out when they get a diagnosis. There is certainly merit to that appellation, but such a hopeful characterization can have unintended consequences. When I told people about my diagnosis, they seemed to sigh with relief that it was only prostate cancer, as if they didn't take it seriously. I came to call it "cancer with training wheels" because it felt like so many people viewed prostate cancer as a lightweight version of the real thing. Make no mistake, though, prostate cancer is no joke: It's the second leading cause of cancer death among males, claiming an American man every 18 minutes. Cure rates, as my surgeon explained, are high because screening has become so effective, resulting in more and more early diagnoses. Catch a tumor when it's confined to the prostate and has a manageable

Gleason score of 6 (I'll explain Gleason scores later in the book), and you're nearly guaranteed a good outcome. But detect it later when the Gleason score is a gnarly 8 or higher and the disease has spread to the bones or other organs, and it's just as deadly as any other cancer. That's the part you don't hear so much about.

Still, prostate cancer does have very high cure rates and, thank God, there are numerous treatment options for men who must grapple with it. Whether you choose radiation, surgery, or focal therapy, there is an abundance of technologies, facilities, and specialists from which to choose. So, yes, I'd rather get a prostate cancer diagnosis than countless other forms of cancer. But that doesn't mean it isn't terrifying to get the call and realize you are now a card-carrying member of the Cancer Club. Until you hear from the doctor that your cancer is eradicated and your PSA is undetectable, the idea that you have the "good cancer" is cold comfort indeed. The best way I've learned to deal with the terror of a cancer diagnosis is to hear how other people coped with the disease, and to address with brutal frankness those aspects of the treatment and recovery process that are often omitted from polite conversation and upbeat websites. If some of the details I share in this book seem graphic or gratuitous, they will not be to men who have similar experiences in their own treatment and recovery. Those are the details I wish someone had shared with me.

I should emphasize that the experiences I recount in this book are based on my having chosen a laparoscopic prostatectomy as my course of treatment. Many men, like my brother-in-law, choose radiation as their first line of defense. Because radiation leaves the prostate intact, the issue of anejaculation is avoided altogether, making it an appealing option for some men. What's more, men who undergo radiation therapy may have fewer potency and incontinence issues, at least initially. Side effects from radiation sometimes appear as much as a year after therapy. Also, radiation permanently changes the tissue in your prostate, making any subsequent surgery very difficult to perform (though not impossible—Sloan Kettering has pioneered what's called the "salvage radical prostatectomy," which is pursued when a rising post-radiation PSA level calls for surgical removal of the prostate gland) and laden with side effects. For some men, like me, who anticipate needing radiation as a second course of treatment, surgery can be the most prudent choice. Focal therapies, which include such exotic-sounding procedures as focal cryoablation and high-intensity focused ultrasound, are minimally invasive options for men with small, localized tumors. By the time we found my tumor, focal therapies were not an option; but for some men they represent a path forward with fewer side effects than radiation or surgery.

Because I have no direct experience with radiation and know only what I read or discussed with the MSK radiation oncologist, I have deliberately given the subject short shrift in this memoir. That is some other guy's book to write. The decision of surgery versus radiation is a huge one. Surgeons, of course, favor surgery, radiation oncologist favor radiation; and both will make a compelling case for their respective approaches. But any reputable doctor will acknowledge that every case of prostate cancer—and I mean *every* one—is unique. As I explain later in this book, treatment decisions must take into account an entire array of data points—Gleason score, staging, PSA level, size and location of the malignancy, MRI results, the patient's age and overall health. In all my research, reading, and discussions, I learned one reliable truth about prostate cancer: Your case is unlike anyone else's. Treat it that way, no matter how tempting it may be to follow the advice of your buddy Tom who had prostate cancer two years ago and was delighted with his proton beam therapy. Nobody, I found, is more persuasive than a successfully treated patient. But for all their well-intended advice, friends and family members who had prostate cancer can only speak to their cases—not to yours. That's between you and your doctor.

1

RANDOM ACTS OF SCREENING

I HATE GETTING PHYSICALS. Ever since I had some bizarre and undiagnosed neurological symptoms thirteen years ago, the specter of which haunted me as doctors struggled to diagnose them, I developed a case of dread about annual exams. Not so with dentists, orthopedists, or optometrists. I just hate the notion that once a year someone looks over my aging body and records the relative rate of decline since the last exam. Blood pressure on the rise. Cholesterol tenaciously high. A touch of osteoarthritis in the shoulder and lower back. The "degenerative cascade," painted in living color, right there on your medical chart. As a result I've tended to procrastinate on scheduling physicals—not in any egregious way. I rarely miss a year, but I don't hurry in when the reminder postcard arrives in the mail, either.

The good news is that my primary care physician, Daniel Quinn, is a great person. I've known him for twenty-five years and we share perspectives on a host of subjects. He supported me when I resisted going on statins for my high cholesterol, recognizing that I didn't have any other factors that suggested I was at risk for heart disease. Instead, he put me on red yeast rice, the natural compound from which some statins were developed, and monitored my progress toward a healthy LDL/HDL ratio. He was measured and reasonable, never pushing me to take antibiotics or strong painkillers, always keeping me calm when I tilted toward hypochondria after doing Internet "research" on a mysterious symptom. Like many physicians, he had read the research on PSA tests and false positives, and elected to use digital rectal exams for prostate cancer screening, reserving PSAs as a follow-up to abnormal findings.

PSA (prostate-specific antigen) tests became popular in the 1990s and were believed to be a useful tool in identifying prostate malignancies before they become problematic—but the tests also had a tendency to produce false positives, or to prompt unnecessary treatment. False positives (test results that were erroneously high) meant that men who didn't have prostate cancer often went rushing in to get re-tested or even have biopsies, only to learn that they had been cancer-free all along. Subsequent research, most notably that of the PLCO (Prostate, Lung, Colorectal, and Ovarian Cancer Screening Trial) and ERSPC (European Randomized Study of Screening for Prostate Cancer) studies published in 2009, cast doubt on whether PSA screening actually reduced death rates at all. Consequently, PSA tests became the subject of considerable public controversy, and skeptical physicians like Dr. Quinn who didn't want to alarm patients with dubious screenings stuck (pun intended) to digital rectal exams as their go-to strategy.

DREs, as these exams are affectionately called, are well-known to men over 50, and the stuff of countless guffaws at Saturday morning golf outings. Generally speaking, the DRE involves having the patient drop his drawers and "assume the position" wherein he squats, boxers bunched around his ankles, as the doctor inserts a gloved and lubricated index finger into his rectum. The prostate gland happens to sit just in front of the rectum, so this point of entry gives the doctor a good feel for the shape and texture of the object in question—though, notably, not all of it. It's an uncomfortable, though generally painless, few seconds for the patient (my wife observes, justifiably, that it doesn't compare to an internal exam at her OB/GYN) leaving him with a lubed-up anus and a phantom sensation of a finger probing the circumference of his poop-shoot. Still, the DRE yields instant results and is over quickly. As a distraction, Dr.

Quinn liked to mention his least favorite politician as his finger eased around my insides. "That way, when you hear his name," he would chuckle, "you'll have the proper association." All this to direct my focus away from the uncomfortable reality that his index finger was three inches inside my rear end.

After it was over, he'd snap the blue glove off his hand, toss it in the trash, and say something like, "Your prostate is smooth, symmetrical, and pliable. No suspicious nodules or irregularities." I'd wipe myself with the Kleenex he provided, zip up my trousers, and gather whatever handouts the nurse had provided. At least that's how it usually went. On this particular appointment, in late October, 2017, I was aware it would be my last exam with Dr. Quinn. He was retiring the following January after forty or so years in practice. As the exam was winding up, he said to me, "Did you have blood taken before your appointment?" I confirmed that I had.

"Good. Then I'm going to suggest that we run a PSA test this time—just to get a baseline number for the future."

I asked him why, and he explained that he had recently overcome his skepticism regarding PSAs and had himself tested. The results came back high, leading to a second test that was also high, then a biopsy, and eventually a diagnosis of prostate cancer. Given the outcome, he decided, it would be prudent to urge his male patients over 50 to take the same precaution. Sure, doing so might yield some false positives, he observed, but erroneous results could be eliminated easily by re-testing. If he caught even one malignancy, he added gravely, it would be worth it. This made perfect sense to me, so I agreed without giving it another thought. After all, we had just finished another annual DRE that signaled everything was okay downtown. My doctor had the nurse call over to the lab to add a PSA to the cholesterol, triglyceride, and other routine tests they would run.

The next morning, I was still in bed at 8 AM, taking my time getting up as I'd come to do since I stopped working full-time the previous year. My cell phone came alive on the bedside table and I grabbed it, answering groggily.

"Hi Jim, this is Pam from Dr. Quinn's office. The doctor asked me to give you a call because your PSA came back high, and Dr.

Amani would like to have you come back in to discuss it." Dr. Desiree Amani was taking over for Dr. Quinn as he eased into retirement. The news broke so quickly I didn't have time to process it.

"How high was it?"

"15.4, which is pretty high," she responded. She went on to explain that anything over a 2 got their attention. So I scheduled to come back in that Monday. Of course, now I had the entire weekend standing between me and additional information, which is never good. I had no real perspective on PSA numbers. One friend of mine, I recalled, had been tested with a PSA of around 4, which had concerned his doctor enough to get him in for a biopsy. It ultimately revealed a malignancy.

So, as any modern medical consumer would do, I grabbed my laptop and checked out various websites using search terms like "Is a PSA of 15.4 high?" and "PSA scores and risk levels." As it turns out, prostate cancer is so common that there are hundreds of useful—and not-so-useful—sites out there to help you interpret every data point associated with the disease. Several sites provided what appeared to be a standardized Prostate Cancer Risk Calculator, which estimates your odds of having cancer based on urinary symptoms or your PSA score. Given what I'd heard about PSA tests and prostate cancer, I figured anyone's odds of having cancer based on a PSA score were ridiculously low. After all, you have to factor in all those false positives. There were typically two calculators. The first asks questions about your general health and urinary habits and gives you a percentage likelihood based on such things as how often you urinate, the strength of your stream and sense of urgency. I answered all the questions honestly and got a score of 6 percent likelihood. That sounded about right. I breathed a sigh of relief.

So I moved on to the second calculator, which bases your odds on an actual PSA test result. I plugged in my number.

Fifty-three percent.

The caption below my score read as follows:

"This risk is the chance (in percent) that prostate cancer will be found if you undergo a prostatic biopsy.

Together with your family physician you can determine whether further examination is desirable."

I didn't exactly freak out when I saw that number, but I did get a hollow feeling deep in my gut. Everyone knows the Internet can convince you that your nasal congestion is actually brain cancer, so I knew to receive this information with a grain of salt. Still, I chose to employ an entire salt shaker in this case. Silently I chastised myself for getting spun up over one number on a standardized risk calculator. However, that didn't stop me from visiting several more websites with calculators. Every score I received was similarly high. At that point, I stepped away from my laptop for the time being. I didn't like how things were trending.

My wife, Barbara, who teaches at nearby Skidmore College, was at work attending her usual Friday department and faculty meetings. I had told her about the high PSA that morning before she left for work. Like me, she took the news with only mild concern, given all we knew about the tests and their unreliability. When she came home early that evening, I told her some of what I had learned online. I caught her a little off-guard. She was just putting down her book bag and purse and heading toward the bathroom when I sprang the 53 percent on her. I felt the cool, outdoor air still lingering on her as she swept by.

"But aren't those tests famously inaccurate?" she asked from inside the powder room. When she emerged, her face was slightly more taut than it had been a moment before. Her concern concerned me.

"Yeah, they are. I'm just surprised they'd give you that high a number right off the bat. I mean, that's a little scary."

She agreed it was alarming, but when I reminded her I was scheduled to see the doctor on Monday, she was reassured. Barbara is all about calmly gathering information and making deeply well-informed decisions. For that reason, her choices are guided by greater foresight than my own. She spares herself needless anxiety by not leaping to conclusions, as I tend to do. I called her deliberate decision-making process "slow cooking" and, though I often chided her for taking too long to act, I couldn't help but admire her discipline. She encouraged me to stay off the Internet over the weekend and reminded me that we had agreed to go to the YMCA that evening for a workout. After my day of worry, 40 sweaty minutes on the elliptical sounded like a helpful distraction.

As she was changing into her workout clothes, Barbara asked if I had happened to call Dr. Quinn to let him know about the results. It had occurred to me, I told her, but his receptionist said, because he was retiring in January, he wasn't taking any new appointments and was honoring only those he had scheduled previously. Barbara reminded me that Daniel was an old friend and wouldn't mind a phone call at his home. So before we left for the Y, I gave him a ring and got his voicemail. I left a brief message alluding to my PSA results and asked him to give me a call at his convenience. After I hung up, I imagined his wife casually checking voicemail before they went out for dinner. So much for HIPAA privacy.

A couple hours later we were leaving the Y after an exhilarating workout when my phone rang. It was Dr. Quinn. He was his usual kind, patient self, his voice just the slightest bit hoarse as if from too many years of reassuring anxious patients. He listened intently to my story, sensing, I'm sure, my growing concern.

"Jim, this is something to take seriously but not to worry about. It could well be a lab error. So I'd wait a couple weeks and get re-tested to see if the number has come down. It could also be related to an infection in your prostate or something else. PSA levels aren't unique to prostate cancer."

I was taking frantic mental notes as he continued: "If the next test comes back high, you'll want to see a urologist. I can recommend a couple here in town who are good. If your urologist recommends a biopsy, I'd try to get an MRI first as an overlay to the biopsy ultrasound. You'll get a more accurate biopsy that way. That's what I did. But insurance doesn't cover it, so you may have to pay like $600 out of pocket. It's worth it, though."

He paused there, probably sensing that I was getting worried with all this talk about biopsies.

"But remember, this is most likely a false alarm. That's why you need to get re-tested. I bet it's a lab error." He indulged me for a few minutes of free-flowing Q & A about biopsies, MRIs, and insurance coverage. Mostly, though, I wanted to hear him say it was probably all a big mistake. After I hung up, I told Barbara what had transpired. She nodded approvingly, as if his prognostication fit her own view of things. We drove home and made the most of the weekend.

Mercifully, my follow-up appointment with Dr. Amani was at 9:15 AM on Monday. So after some cereal and an exceptionally large cup of coffee from the local Stewart's Shop convenience store, I made the short drive to the doctor's office. Moments later, I was in an examination room meeting with Dr. Amani, an attractive ebony-skinned woman with a lilting African accent. I'd met her a couple of other times when Dr. Quinn wasn't available, and had been impressed with her manner. She explained all the vagaries of PSA testing, repeating much of what Dr. Quinn said on Friday. She, too, recommended getting re-tested and gave me the names of two local urologists. Wary of unnecessary invasive procedures, I asked whether a specialist was likely to push me toward a premature biopsy. She was confident any urologist would want a second PSA before moving to a biopsy.

Dr. Amani was aware I had developed a wicked case of anxiety shortly after I left my job as a senior executive at a marketing firm. In fact, it was Amani who met with me to discuss my initial symptoms—tightness in the chest, shallow breathing, sense of impending doom, visions of the apocalypse, that sort of thing—and who wrote a 30-day prescription for Klonopin, which turned out to be miraculous in quieting my turbulent mind. I'm sure my anxiety was on her mind as we spoke about the PSA results. Either that or I was giving her the deer-in-headlights look that makes doctors slow down and speak carefully.

"You know," she said with her beautiful accent and a penetrating look, "we call prostate cancer the 'good cancer' because if you have to get cancer, this is the one to get."

I smiled wanly.

"The cure rates are very, very high." Then she paused again and added, "But let's hope this is something else."

At that moment, an idea popped into my head. "You know, I've ridden horses for about ten years, and it involves a lot of pounding on my groin area. Do you think it's possible I inflamed my prostate somehow and it affected my test?"

"Yes, it very well could have," she replied, seizing on my need to find an alternate etiology. "When you talk to the urologist, you should mention that because he may ask you not to ride between now and your next test." I was smiling inside now. That was it: All those years of cantering around the ring and leaping over fences had aggravated my prostate, and the PSA levels were nothing more than an admonition to ease up on the riding. Somewhere in my mind a slender ray of sunlight appeared through parting clouds.

Clinging to this alternative narrative, I dutifully called around to urologists in Saratoga. That was a memorable experience. My first call was to a urologist I'd seen years before to have a varicocele repaired. For the record, and to demonstrate that I have an apparent proclivity for seeking out surgery involving my genitals, varicocele repair is a procedure to eliminate an enlarged vein in your scrotum. Apparently these veins can raise the temperature around your testicles and cause low sperm production. Back when Barbara and I were having difficulty getting pregnant, I sought this urologist to correct the problem. The procedure went beautifully—and provided absolutely no discernible benefit other than to give me an impressive scar where no one but my wife will ever see it. In any case, I called this doctor to set an appointment. The woman who answered was young and officious, an attitude I recognized by how she answered the phone: hurried and slightly irritated to be distracted from whatever she was working on. I calmly explained that I had been a patient of Dr. X years ago, and recently had a PSA score of 15.4, so I wanted to make an appointment.

"I should tell you that Dr. X is currently scheduling into April of next year," she replied, unfazed by my PSA. I felt like I was supposed to congratulate Dr. X for having such a land-office business.

"Really? There isn't any way to expedite an appointment, given my circumstances?"

"I can put you on a waiting list," she replied, "but I can't guarantee anything." I could tell she was opening up a calendar to see what she could find in the distant future of Dr. X's prolific revenue stream.

At that point I got angry. Even if she couldn't do better with an appointment, I was stunned that a professional at a urology office wouldn't recognize the significance of a sky-high PSA and show some empathy for the worried man on the phone.

The whole subject of empathy and medical professionals' ability to exhibit it became a theme in my treatment. I came to view that single characteristic as perhaps the most important ingredient in caregiving. At Memorial Sloan Kettering I witnessed the inspiring example of an organization that had institutionalized empathy so effectively that one felt compassion in every encounter—from the surgeon to the phlebotomist to the receptionist. Elsewhere, however, I saw a troubling and pervasive absence of empathy where you would expect to find it most—at local specialists' practices and, perhaps most disappointing, our hometown hospital emergency room.

"No, don't bother," I responded abruptly. "There are plenty of urologists in the world. I'll find one that can make time for urgent matters." I hung up before she could respond. I was steaming. Maybe I'd been too quick to cut her off, but I was feeling emotionally raw and wasn't prepared to be snubbed by the very profession to which I needed access.

I called another number I'd been provided by Dr. Amani, with no success, and then turned to the Web for names and reviews of leading urologists in the Capital District (the larger metropolitan area beyond Saratoga Springs, including Albany, Schenectady, and Troy). As expected, there was an abundance of urologists. Reviews from sources like Google and HealthGrades helped me winnow the list down and I started dialing. One fellow I came across was located in Albany on the campus of St. Peter's Hospital. His reviews were strong and he had impressive credentials in urologic oncology—though I hoped like hell the oncology part would prove irrelevant.

A call to his office put me in touch with a very nice woman at the front desk. She indicated that, though Dr. Z was booked up, she would refer my information to him right away and, because my PSA was elevated, he would likely make time to see me in the coming week. *That's more like it,* I thought. Sure enough, the next day I got a call from Dr. Z's office. He could see me on Monday, November 6.

Dr. Z turned out to be a nice enough man. He was short, black-haired, athletically built, and meticulously groomed. He exuded confidence, referencing all the latest studies on PSAs and standards of care, signaling to me that he took his research and his outcomes very, very seriously. He had a nice way of being direct without being blunt, and answered my questions thoughtfully. He spoke of a consultative approach to diagnosis and treatment. Patients and doctors should work together to develop a plan, he said. As expected, he recommended re-testing. "Did you prep for your last PSA test?" he asked.

This was a surprise. I knew to fast for cholesterol tests but had no idea one prepared for a PSA test. I asked for details.

"Well, basically you avoid doing anything that might aggravate your prostate, so no bicycle or horseback riding for a week before. And no sex for 48 hours before. That can raise your PSA slightly as well." This was all news to me, raising the brief hope that my high score was due to a lack of preparation. As he spoke, though, I recalled that, for about two weeks prior to my first PSA I hadn't been riding my horse, so I would have met the standards for "prepping." Damn. Perhaps, though, the *long-term* trauma to my prostate had left me with a deceptively high PSA. This kind of rationalizing with myself became a constant dynamic in my treatment. The more the data concerned me, the more impressive my mental gymnastics became to reshape my reality.

Dr. Z also indicated that he was ordering a more specific test, one that measured both PSA and "free PSA." He explained that the prostate-specific antigen circulates through the body in two ways: either bound to other proteins or on its own. The relative levels of each could tell us more than the PSA test alone. When I went home to learn more about free PSA, I read on the Harvard Medical School Prostate Knowledge website that doctors will often order a free PSA test for men with a number between 4 and 10 ng/ml, which is considered a "gray area" for PSA scores. Obviously I didn't fit this category, but I liked that Dr. Z was doing it anyway. Men in this zone who have a free PSA greater than 25 percent are more likely to have a benign condition and not cancer, which rules out the need for a biopsy. All this was encouraging to me. My constantly-revising narrative required there be lots of open questions about my high score. The more uncertainty, the better.

My re-test was scheduled. I would have blood drawn at an urgent care center in Saratoga and would receive the results from Dr. Z on December 11. In the meantime, I set about pampering my prostate by avoiding bicycles and horses and even going easy on the elliptical machine at the Y. I took care to seat myself gently on hard surfaces and didn't strain on the toilet. I followed advice Dr. Z never gave me, but this prostate was going to be so lovingly protected that whatever aberration led to a 15.4 was going away in a jiffy. With every passing day, I became more confident that the first test had been either a lab error or was picking up on my prostate-unfriendly equestrian lifestyle. Further encouraging me was the fact that I had none of the urinary symptoms associated with prostate cancer. Relatively strong urine flow (for a 56 year-old, at least), no need to urinate frequently, no real urgency when I had to go. Plus, I had years of good DRE results from Dr. Quinn. Even Dr. Z agreed that these were good signs.

On a trip to New York City during November, I developed some odd symptoms in my lower back, abdomen, and groin. My back ached as if someone had punched me in my kidneys. On top of that, I felt swollen lymph nodes in my armpits and the back of my neck. I even had pain in my groin and perineum, which struck me as particularly relevant. Convinced this array of symptoms indicated an infection, I called Dr. Z to share the news, expecting to hear, "Ah, okay, this explains a lot. I think you've got a mild infection of the prostate. I'm writing you a script for an antibiotic."

I left a message with his receptionist and he called me back when I was walking along Central Park West on the way to midtown. When I saw his number on my caller ID, I ducked into the park where I could talk more privately. Dr. Z was obviously calling between patients and sounded slightly harassed. After hearing my litany of symptoms, he asked if I had any blood in my urine. No, I replied. Any pain when you urinate? No. Any pain when you ejaculate? No.

Long pause.

"My best guess is these symptoms are unrelated," he explained. "As for the pain in your kidney area, I can schedule a renal scan to see what's going on there. But I don't think any of this has to do with your PSA."

I've never been so disappointed to hear that I *didn't* have a prostate infection. Days later, as if disarmed by the doctor's assessment of their significance, most of my symptoms mysteriously subsided. The "kidney" pain, I later decided, came from "Russian twists," a core exercise I was fond of for my oblique and lower back muscles. The groin pain probably came from overdoing "come-togethers," which work the muscles in the lower abdomen. As for the swollen lymph nodes, I might have been fighting a virus. It was, after all, flu season. I couldn't explain the feelings in my perineum and never did.

Reflecting on my psychological processing of the cancer experience, I'm struck by how the human mind can construct a narrative where one might be unavailable, incomplete, or unsatisfying. Where tidy certainty is elusive, our overzealous imaginations provide an alternative reality, cobbled together from otherwise unremarkable physical symptoms. My various aches and pains were all (or mostly) real, but my subconscious rearranged and connected them into a fanciful diagnosis of a prostate infection, or contusion, or anything but cancer. Once I realized my mind was playing tricks on me, I admonished myself for allowing it to happen. The whole thing made me feel like a hypochondriac.

Having given this puzzling phenomenon a great deal of thought, however, I've taken a different view, which is that we have a wonderful capacity for self-protection and self-comforting. None of the alternative narratives my mind produced played out, but there were moments when they pacified the anxiety raging inside me; and surely that was of value. None of these flights of fancy altered my course of action, resulted in procrastination, or made me resistant to the truth when I learned it. I still ended up at Sloan Kettering for a five-hour surgery as scheduled and went through all the experiences my imagination tried to rule out. But my travels toward that moment were made more tolerable at times by the belief that, for example, I had an infection or had traumatized my prostate by riding. That we are beings, conscious of and tormented by our own mortality, is a curse. That we can willfully alter our conscious experience of reality to soothe ourselves is, I have decided, a blessing.

When December 11 rolled around, I was a confused mix of confident and terrified, my psyche operating on two emotional levels. My confidence felt like an intellectual overlay I had constructed to protect myself from fear. It was a narrative of selectively assembled facts from test results, reading, conversations with doctors, and physical sensations. The other, deeper psychological stratum was doubtful and vulnerable, but also coldly rational, and keenly aware that the universe is a random environment in which there is no coherent teleology, no long arc toward justice. Things happen for no good reason, and that's that. Over time I learned that these two layers would always be present, constantly bumping into and revising each other on the shifting, turbulent plain of my consciousness.

As she had done previously, the nurse recorded my vital signs before the doctor came in. Then a few quiet minutes passed before I heard the soft shuffling of Dr. Z's Crocs in the hallway, then the opening of the door. He came in with the same hurried but casual air of confidence. Without even saying hello, he looked me squarely in the face and said, "Well, your PSA is still high. And the free PSA number didn't clear anything up for me."

None of this came across as abrupt or rude. I think he appreciated that I wanted to hear the facts as quickly as possible, and pleasantries would only defer the moment of truth. Thus far, his approach had been fine with me. We talked for a few minutes about what my PSA score meant. He referred to my number as being "convincingly high," a phrase I came to dislike for its ominous implications. At this point, I could feel some of the open questions, the alternative etiologies for my high PSA, evaporating like raindrops on a hot sidewalk. When I obliquely referred to my number as having stayed the same, he corrected me.

"To be clear, Jim, your number actually went up. It's now

19.6. So we don't like that too much."

No shit, I thought, responding with muted hostility to his use of the plural pronoun. But I checked my momentary frustration and continued to listen. Given the fact that my number was high and had actually moved up substantially—a concept referred to as "velocity"—in a few weeks, he did not think continued monitoring of my PSA was a viable option, nor did he believe I would embrace that choice. Instead, he recommended we conduct a biopsy to see what was going on down there. The word "biopsy" cued memories of my conversation with Dr. Quinn in which he strongly recommended an MRI (magnetic resonance imaging, a machine that employs powerful magnets to take detailed images of your interior) to help guide the biopsy process. I ran the idea by Dr. Z, explaining that my primary care physician had done the same thing to diagnose his own prostate cancer. This is where Dr. Z's tone shifted slightly but perceptibly. While his answers still focused on the collaborative approach to setting a treatment plan, I could tell he resisted the MRI idea. His answers became subtly evasive, and I sensed a rigidity in his rationale. We went back and forth, with me pushing more and more for the MRI and him indicating it wasn't appropriate at this point. I explained I'd be willing to pay out of pocket if necessary. He came closest to agreeing when he remarked with a hint of condescension, "Well, it's not a standard of care and not something I would recommend, but if it would give you peace of mind, we can explore that option." Was he accusing me of being a hypochondriac or an alarmist? I bristled at this change in tone. I pushed some more and then, eventually, perhaps out of weariness and a desire just to get some resolution, I acquiesced, agreeing to proceed with the standard ultrasound biopsy. We agreed to keep the MRI as an option to investigate biopsy results if necessary. His answers that day never sat well with me. It felt like I was hearing the insurance company's voice coming through, a nuance that marked the beginning of my faltering confidence in Dr. Z.

Scheduling any medical procedure during the holidays is always a challenge. Fortunately, Dr. Z performed biopsies in his office on designated days each week, so we started looking at dates right away. I told him I'd like to get the biopsy over with as soon as possible, so our family's holiday wouldn't be shrouded by uncertainty. To my surprise, he rearranged his schedule to fit me in that coming Thursday, only three days later. The procedure, he said, takes about an hour and would require that someone drive me to and from the appointment. I booked the time slot, received a handful of instructions for the biopsy prep, and headed for home, feeling substantially less confident in my carefully-wrought narrative than I had before hearing my new PSA score.

2

MERRY CHRISTMAS

PRIOR TO HAVING PROSTATE CANCER, my experience with biopsies had largely been limited to removing "suspicious" moles at the dermatologist. My wife Barbara had a more serious biopsy experience when her OB/GYN detected a nodule on her thyroid gland. Concerned that the bump might be malignant, her doctor ordered an ultrasound-guided needle biopsy. I remember going with Barbara to her appointment and trying to calm her as she contemplated the idea of a needle plunging into the hard center of her arched neck. Sure enough, the experience was every bit as uncomfortable as she expected. Being with her at that appointment made an impression on me. I would have hated it just as much as my wife did. Barbara is the first to admit that she's queasy about needles. She's the kind of patient who, when the phlebotomist readies the syringe to take blood, looks anywhere but at her arm and talks animatedly about any subject that pops into her mind—all to distract herself. In contrast, I saw myself as relatively laid-back about most medical procedures (except, later in life, physicals), having shown admirable toughness, I believed, during four colonoscopies, an array of broken bones, a varicocele repair, and stitches in my cheek and shin. Blood didn't freak me out and needles were generally manageable. However, I was now having significant misgivings about a procedure that involved large needles deep inside my rear end.

For one thing, I had a hard time envisioning how prostate biopsies are conducted. The whole process seemed so difficult to carry off. I knew they used a rectal probe that employs ultrasound imaging to guide the biopsy needle, which carefully (and, I hoped, gently) punches holes through the rectum into the neighboring prostate. The idea was to obtain about a dozen "cores" of prostate tissue from different parts of the gland. Doing so gives a broad perspective on the extent of any malignancy. Once gathered, the tissue samples are sent to a pathologist who reviews them under a microscope and provides a written report on whether cancer is present, how developed it is, and where in the prostate it is located. Pathologists can determine all this based on which of the core samples contain cancerous cells and what percentage of each is cancerous versus healthy tissue. My ideal pathology report, of course, would be some version of "All we found is healthy prostate tissue. Go home and have a beer."

When I scheduled my biopsy, Dr. Z's nurse gave me a handout titled "Prostate Biopsy and Ultrasound: About This Test." It featured an illustrated cross-section of a lower abdomen, complete with a penis, testicles, and anus—all neatly halved for inspection. The picture showed an ultrasound probe inserted into the rectum with a biopsy needle protruding from it like a tiny bayonet. The probe looked bigger than Dr. Quinn's finger, which was my only point of reference for this sort of thing— about the circumference of a Corona cigar. A second, more detailed illustration showed how the biopsy needle extended into the prostate, aimed directly at a small white area inside the gland labeled "mass." I wondered whether "mass" was intended as euphemism or meant to suggest that something other than cancer could be found growing inside your prostate. I tended toward the former.

In the days leading up to the biopsy, I was told to discontinue any supplements or medications that could thin my blood, such as aspirin or fish oil. I was also told to purchase a Fleet enema and use it the night before the biopsy to clear any fecal matter from my colon. If any such matter shows up at the party, the doctor warned me, the party is canceled and everyone goes home. I believe I was told to lay off food for a while before the procedure. I don't recall those details. I was too focused on the fact that, between the enema and the ultrasound probe, I'd have two foreign objects stuck up my rear in the space of twelve hours.

The nurse told me I could buy the enema at any local pharmacy, but I was strongly inclined to order one online. Because I live in a small town, it's not unusual to encounter a friend or business acquaintance at the drugstore, and I could only imagine the awkward moment when an ex-employee, clutching some cough syrup and a bag of chips, got in line behind me as the LED display on the cash register flashed, "Enema for the old guy." This was to be avoided at any cost. However, given how soon the ultrasound was scheduled, I couldn't be assured my package would arrive on time from Amazon. So instead, I chose a Rite-Aid on the outskirts of town and took my chances. As luck would have it, I couldn't find the green and white Fleet enema box and was forced to ask the chipper woman behind the pharmacy counter for guidance. My cover blown, I thanked her, took a "2-Pack" (in case the first pack didn't work out) from the shelf, and warily proceeded to the checkout.

As I stood in line, my mind played back a fragment from T. S. Eliot's Prufrock: "I have seen the moment of my greatness flicker, / And I have seen the eternal Footman hold my coat, and snicker . . . " Eliot started writing that poem when he was only 22. How the hell did he understand so well what it felt like to buy an enema at Rite-Aid? Mercifully, the cashier went about her job so automatically she scarcely looked at me, much less took the time to snicker. Even so, my masculine greatness already felt extinguished as I ducked into my car and headed home with a two-pack of enemas and a growing sense of dread.

The enema was interesting. The Fleet product is just a plastic bottle full of sodium phosphates, a solution that works by drawing water into the colon "to rapidly produce a bowel movement." It has a long, soft rubber applicator on the business end covered by a protective plastic wrap. The instructions say to lie on your side in the fetal position, insert the enema in your rectum, squeeze the bottle until the liquid is nearly gone, and wait a few minutes for the action to start. My first dilemma was where I would go to perform such a procedure. Given the desired outcome, I chose the bathroom floor, on which I spread a clean towel over the cold ceramic tiles. I was tempted to light a few candles and play some Enya music, but that seemed indulgent. I can't say exactly when in my cancer journey my dignity began to falter, but this was certainly a milestone. I hadn't been this intimate with a bathroom floor since an unfortunate interaction with tequila on my twenty-first birthday. Following the enema instructions with grave intensity, I curled up, braced myself, and inserted the rubber applicator. For all my apprehensiveness, the insertion was a non-event; and the sensation of water shooting up my rear wasn't so uncomfortable, either. The good thing about enemas, I learned, is that they work really fast. The instructions said I should experience a bowel movement in two to five minutes, so I had my watch handy to tick off the minutes to countdown, but there was no need for such formalities. Almost immediately, pressure started to build in my abdomen as if a Nerf football was working its way through my colon. Caught off-guard by how quickly the Fleet took effect, I sprang to my feet and on to the toilet just seconds before the magic happened. No more than ninety seconds after the fateful insertion, I stood up feeling deliriously empty and squeaky clean. Fleet enemas, it turns out, don't mess around.

The next morning, my wife drove me the 30 miles to Dr. Z's office in Albany. Neither of us was feeling particularly chipper so we talked quietly, allowing long pauses between subjects. At the doctor's office, Barbara took her place in the waiting room, settling in with a book and notepaper to catch up on her class preparation. Meanwhile, I gave a urine sample as usual and proceeded to the biopsy room where the equipment was assembled. The machines were clean and white with various electrical cords and tubes coiled up tidily like braids on a general's shoulder. There was a large video monitor through which, I presumed, the doctor would see my prostate and guide the needle. There may have been a joystick, though that could have been my imagination. To avoid any infection arising from poking holes in a space reserved for fecal evacuation, Dr. Z prescribed an antibiotic that I took days before and immediately following the biopsy. He also gave me a single Valium tablet to help me relax during the procedure. I was instructed to take it forty-five minutes before we began. I had never taken a Valium, or at least not that I remembered, but looking back on the biopsy, I can confirm that Valium is an exceptionally good idea. By the time I had removed my clothes and was donning my gown, I felt a pleasant, woozy sensation creeping through my body. The drug didn't make me feel disoriented or sloppy. Rather, it relaxed every muscle, every joint, every nerve, right down to my molecular structure. By the time I had my hospital gown on, I was one extremely chill customer. Of course, knowing what I know now, I would have preferred a handful of Valiums—or better yet, to be knocked out entirely.

The Valium may account for my fuzzy memory of the procedure. Once on the examination table, I assumed the fetal position again (there must be an appropriate metaphor for why older men with prostate cancer curl up like fetuses so often, but I haven't figured that one out). A cold topical anesthetic was applied in my rear end, and then the probe made its appearance, though I didn't see it. It must have been one of those items coiled up by the video monitor. Dr. Z had explained that he would take about a dozen cores and that, each time he did so, the nurse assisting him would review the quality of the core and call out "Okay." If the core wasn't satisfactory, she would say, "No," at which point they would try again. The objective was to get good samples from all different parts of the prostate, so they would be moving the probe into position before each needle stick. "You're going to hear a loud 'click' each time we take a core," Dr. Z said. "Don't be alarmed by that."

Several years earlier, I had decided to have some body hair removed from my back and shoulders. I had just enough that it made me self-conscious at the beach or swimming pool. For the record, we're talking sparse follicular groves on the deltoids and trapezius, not a dense forest of back hair like some men I've seen in the Y locker room. I had an excellent dermatologist who recommended laser hair removal as an effective and permanent solution. She warned me, however, that each burst of laser light can smart—like having a rubber band snapped against your skin over and over again. It was a good comparison and, sure enough, that's what it felt like. It hurt enough to elicit a grimace each time the laser flashed, but it was manageable. In contrast, Dr. Z had no such analogy for this procedure. Left to my own devices, I imagined a needle stick like a flu shot: a brief prick, some slight stinging, and then it would be over. Here's why that assumption was wrong: The biopsy needle removes a small core of tissue from your prostate, so it is larger and meaner than your routine flu shot needle. Additionally, the needle shoots out of a probe, through the wall of the rectum itself, and into the adjacent gland. That's a lot of tissue and nerves to mess with. And in case the needle stick didn't get my attention, the "click" Dr. Z referred to turned out to be a baritone, hollow-sounding *chock* that echoed around the room like a broken snare drum.

The first time I heard *chock* and felt the needle stick, I nearly vaulted off the table. The needle felt big and dull and hit with surprising force—not at all like a flu shot. In my astonishment and pain, I let go a couple loud expletives. "I know," said Dr. Z, "It hurts. I'm sorry. Hang in there. How was that one, Kim?"

"Good," the nurse responded.

Then he maneuvered the probe from side to side, aiming at a different spot.

Chock.

Pause.

"Good."

Pressure and pain inside my rear end as the probe is repositioned.

Chock.

"Good."

"Just a few more, now."

Each time the needle did its thing, I wondered to myself, *why didn't anyone tell me how much this would hurt? Or why didn't they just knock me out?* The illustration on my handout looked harmless enough. But this hurt like hell. All told, I believe the probe was inside me for only ten minutes. Dr. Z moved quickly and purposefully, at times maneuvering the probe forcefully to achieve a particular angle he needed. Each of the needle sticks hurt just like the first one, and the snare-drum reminders didn't help me find my inner peace. But then, mercifully, it was over. The doctor cleaned me up, tossing some bloody gauze squares onto a tray by the table, and told me I could get dressed. There was a dull pain throbbing in my rear, but it was already beginning to fade. As I pulled on my pants, I asked sheepishly if other men complain about the pain.

"Oh, yeah," he said. "I've actually recommended that we change the standard of care to general anesthesia. But that hasn't been adopted yet."

That's because, I thought to myself, *urologists aren't the ones lying on a table in the fetal position having this devil needle go at them over and over again.*

I was advised to take it easy for the next couple of days. "You may have blood in your stool and semen for a while," said Dr. Z, to which I raised an eyebrow. "It's totally normal. The blood in your stool should pass pretty quickly," he said. "It might take longer for the semen to return to normal."

I asked when the biopsy results would be available. It was close to Christmas and I didn't want the uncertainty to cast a pall over our holiday. The results would be available in seven to ten days, but Dr. Z offered to push the pathologist to get back to us by the end of the following week. We scheduled our follow-up appointment for Friday the 22nd, the same day my daughter Mattie was coming home for Christmas.

The week after my biopsy was a busy time. Barbara frantically graded exams so she wouldn't have a lot of work over the holiday. We did our remaining Christmas shopping. The weather was unrelentingly cold and cloudy. I was a little sore from the needle sticks but that improved quickly. As predicted, my next few bowel movements showed black blood in the stool. It was visually disturbing, but I was glad to have been warned about it. More alarming was what Dr. Z described as "some blood" in my semen. There didn't seem to be anything *other* than blood—old, dark blood the color of prune juice. That particular phenomenon took a couple weeks to resolve itself and I was mighty relieved when it did.

My appointment on the 22nd was at 9 AM. Barbara insisted on going with me, and I welcomed her company with gratitude. As each phase of this process unfolded, I found myself feeling emotionally wobbly and, unexpectedly, willing to confide my vulnerability to my wife. Knowing Barbara was just as stressed as I was, I didn't want to burden her unduly, but I also knew she appreciated when we could talk with complete honesty. As with a lot of men, sharing my deepest feelings wasn't generally my M.O., so Barbara found my newfound candor refreshing. In turn, I got tremendous relief from talking it all through and being reassured that anyone would be a little freaked out over this. Over time, our conversations were less about "next steps" and what we read on the Internet, and more about how the threat of cancer colored our experience of each day, our outlook, and our interaction with each other. The specter of cancer, ironically, forged a stronger bond between us, even as we occasionally retreated back into ourselves to brood privately. Each of us understood this was fundamentally a shared experience. Neither of us could escape it just as neither of us was facing it alone.

It was my fourth trip to Dr. Z's office, Barbara's second. Because Mattie was arriving in Albany by train that evening, we decided to spend the day shopping at a mall not far from the doctor's office, after which we would go to the train station. Whatever news we received, we were determined to have some fun that day, to claim some small share of holiday spirit. When the nurse called my name at Dr. Z's office, Barbara squeezed my hand and gave me a lingering, reassuring look. I forced a weak smile and followed the nurse out of the reception area. All morning my heart had been thumping violently in my chest and my breathing had been tight and shallow—the usual signs of anxiety. Anticipating I might be a basket case for this meeting, I requested a refill on my Klonopin prescription and popped one of the little yellow miracles before I left the house. Even with the Klonopin, however, I was a shit-storm inside, and when the nurse took my vital signs, my blood pressure was way above normal. She wrote down my numbers, remarking, "A little nervous today?"

I laughed sardonically. Boy, did she miss the mark.

Five minutes might have passed between when the nurse left and Dr. Z came into the room. I sat on a plastic chair in the white hum of the fluorescent lights, practicing my deep breathing: inhale for four seconds, hold for four seconds, exhale for seven seconds. It wasn't working. I was mid-breath when the latch on the door turned and Dr. Z walked in. Before I could say a thing, he gave me a sympathetic smile and said, "Well, we found some cancer, I'm afraid."

And with that, I was instantly altered. With those few words, I went from being an otherwise very healthy man with a curiously elevated PSA to being a cancer patient. It was rather anticlimactic, except for the timpani of my pounding heart. Strangely, the anxiety arose from anticipating the results and began receding with the doctor's lightning-fast disclosure. Dr. Z, who must have delivered similar news to countless men over the years, undoubtedly knew that the agony exists in not knowing, so transmitting the dreaded information as fast as possible was an act of mercy. As we talked through all the implications, I could feel the tension in my body relaxing. Mostly, I regretted that I knew the diagnosis and had, to some extent, been put out of my misery. Barbara, though, was sitting in the reception area, still suffering from the fit of apprehension I had experienced. Now that I knew the outcome, I wanted to tell her as quickly as possible, but there was so much to discuss with the doctor, including treatment options, my Gleason score, the clinical stage of my tumor, and other alluring concepts.

In retrospect, I realize I should have paused the conversation and invited Barbara into the examination room, but some monkey-brain masculine instinct told me to tough it out, as if hearing the news by myself was a mark of strength. Consciously overruling those primitive inclinations became an ongoing exercise during my cancer treatment. Each time I found myself inclined to withdraw inside my masculine self and suffer in silence, I recalled articles my daughter Mattie showed me from her sociology class on gender roles. How often, I wondered, do men deny themselves the tenderness of a loved one's support because they are tyrannized by cultural expectations of what it means to be a man? That was a can of worms I would peek into time and again.

I've heard people say they were shocked when they got their cancer diagnosis, that it couldn't be them, that there must have been a mistake at the pathology lab. I had none of that reaction. In fact, the moment I knew my diagnosis, it felt like it had been the only outcome possible. For all my mental gyrations to convince myself I wasn't sick, it now felt absolutely coherent. *Of course I had cancer*, I thought; my PSA was a sky-high 19.6, not a nicely ambiguous 4. For all my attempts to hammer empirical facts into the "I don't have cancer" narrative, this new story felt strangely providential, bordering on rational. Somehow, that calmed me down.

Dr. Z explained that my pathology results looked overall very encouraging: My Gleason score was a tame 6 (I'll explain this in more detail later, but anything above a Gleason 6 is concerning), and the presence of cancer in only two of the twelve tissues samples suggested my tumor was small. These two data points indicated a cancer that was caught early and should be very curable. "So, that's two happy boxes we can check," Dr. Z said reassuringly. "What I don't like as much is your PSA of 19.6, which suggests there might be something we're not seeing from the biopsy." For that reason he suggested—*wait for it*—an MRI, which would let us view the prostate and its tumor with far greater clarity. You may recall, this was the very procedure I had asked for *before* undertaking my biopsy so we could have more imaging with which to guide the biopsy needle. This was also the procedure Dr. Z had opposed out of obedience, I came to believe, to insurance guidelines. With this development, my confidence in Dr. Z took its first real hit. It wouldn't be the last time. Nonetheless, here we were, so I agreed to the MRI. The doctor had his team schedule me at his preferred imaging provider in nearby Latham. Just before I left, Dr. Z handed me a book, *100 Questions and Answers About Prostate Cancer*. It was a hefty paperback featuring a pastiche of cheesy stock photos on the cover: a wife with her arms flung around her husband's neck, both of them smiling; a devilishly handsome man with his hand resting on his chin, lost in contemplation; and a serious looking African-American man peering deeply into the camera. The book design signaled rampant euphemism. But then I read one of the blurbs on the cover, the clinical coldness of which stopped me in my tracks:

"What are castrate-resistant prostate cancer (CRPC) and metastatic castrate-resistant prostate cancer (mCRPC) and how are they treated?"

That's a hell of a blurb, I mused. *In one sentence it mentions castration and metastasis.* If this was supposed to boost the spirits of a newly diagnosed cancer patient, the publisher might want to reconsider the cover presentation.

"There's a lot of good information in this book," Dr. Z said as he handed it to me. "I strongly recommend looking it over."

As I stood to leave, the nurse came in with a paper on which she had handwritten my Gleason score, my clinical stage, and my most recent PSA score. These three numbers, I learned, were like my cancer credentials. They would be referenced repeatedly in discussions about treatment options, risk of recurrence, and survival rates. With this paper in one hand and my new book in the other, I headed to the receptionist area to schedule my MRI. When I stopped at the desk, I could see into the waiting room where Barbara was sitting. She had spotted me first and her intense blue eyes were locked on me. I had been gone a long time, I realized with regret, and her face registered the anxiety of a person who had endured too much uncertainty. My heart sank just looking at her.

I pursed my lips in disappointment and shook my head from side to side. She cast her eyes down toward her lap where she held a book she'd been trying to read.

Merry Christmas.

3

ALTERED

MANY PEOPLE WHO have had cancer reach a point of saturation with thinking, worrying, talking about the disease. They don't want their daily lives to be consumed by cancer, to be "defined" by it, as I've heard it said. I understand that phenomenon, having had many moments when Barbara and I would call a "time-out" on cancer and move on to less fraught, blissfully mundane subjects. Cancer is profoundly disruptive to the progression of one's life, drawing a demarcation between existence before and existence after the disease first appeared. When I say I was altered by my diagnosis, I mean that in a several ways. Most significantly, there was a new, pervasive worry. Once you've been told there are malignant cells growing inside you, conspiring like prison inmates to break free and wreak havoc on your body, you introduce a permanent uneasiness into your world view. Life, already complicated by middle age, becomes a process of moving forward while constantly looking over your shoulder—a twisted take on the poet Andrew Marvell's "But at my back I always hear / Time's wingéd chariot hurrying near." It's haunting to know that just a few rogue cells left behind by the surgeon's scalpel or the beam of the CyberKnife can mass once again to launch a new assault, hastening the day of your demise. My perspective has been altered by the anticipation of milestones when I receive crucial new information, like the post-surgical pathology report or the six-month PSA test, the outcomes of which can bend the course of my life in unimagined ways. Every piece of encouraging news is qualified, leaving me to anticipate passage through the next gate, and the next, as required permission to advance in life. It makes life a halting affair and shortens the arc of one's perspective.

Cancer and other life-threatening health challenges, it is commonly said, change how a person experiences life: The present takes on more vivid meaning, and enjoyment of life's little pleasures becomes intensified. People become less focused on career and money and more on enjoying the emotionally gratifying aspects of life—watching the sprinkler do its slow work on a hot summer afternoon or tossing a football with your brother. Moments like those still resonate deeply with me, but honestly, cancer hasn't changed my experience of them. At times I almost feel cheated that my illness hasn't resulted in that deeper appreciation of the here and now. Maybe the threat of my prostate cancer wasn't terrifying enough to cause that perspectival reframing. I don't know. Maybe I was always preoccupied with mortality, and cancer just gave me a justification to stay that way. Oddly, it was a feeling similar to my emotions when I bought a house. When Barbara and I were in graduate school renting an apartment, I looked at homeowners my age as having crossed over into an exclusive, adult existence. They knew the secrets of a mortgage and building equity; they felt the responsibility of household budgets and home maintenance projects. When we eventually bought our first home, I felt like I had been initiated into that secret society, and I was proud. Similarly, when I was diagnosed with cancer, the veil over another secret world was lifted—I experienced firsthand the mysterious rites of passage through which cancer patients journey: diagnosis, MRIs, blood tests, surgery, recovery, setbacks, fear, humiliation, anger. I know it sounds strange, but for me it's been a very real dynamic. The gnostic knowledge I have gained, however dearly, has been a kind of recompense for the suffering. Of course, I say that with confidence my life won't be shortened by this disease. It's possible, I suppose, that were I faced with a grim prognosis of only a couple of years to live, I might feel my induction into the Cancer Club, with all its occult knowledge, was insufficient payment for a looming death sentence. I hope never to be forced into making that determination.

Perhaps I so keenly felt that sense of initiation because, like most people in my generation, I never faced a profound existential threat—never had my courage or moral conviction tested in an epoch-defining conflict—and cancer provided some form of that. Our parents' generation had its character forged in the devastation of the Great Depression and World War II. My father was a paratrooper in the 82nd Airborne Division. He jumped out of airplanes into enemy territory, crossed rivers at night under heavy fire, liberated a concentration camp, and saw friends blown to pieces. Those experiences made him, I believe, a stronger, better person. Of course, he had his foibles and failures, but at his core there was a confidence that he could endure the worst life threw at him. And he did, many times. It's not surprising that my father was the first person I wanted to call when I was diagnosed. But he had died from pancreatic cancer several years earlier. Almost every day I learn something about cancer that makes me want to call him. I think he would appreciate some of the firsthand details, though his experiences with cancer were very different. I wonder if he would have recognized a change in me as I mustered my fortitude to meet the challenge, if he would have asked me probing questions about my diagnosis, my surgery, my recovery, my state of mind. In the strange way I have described, I would have been proud to tell him.

There is yet another way I felt changed by cancer. Both my parents died from cancer; and the disease had been such a presence in my life for so long that being diagnosed felt like coming face to face with a distant relative, someone I'd known by reputation but had never met. It was like a dark family reunion. As I wrote earlier, my mother died of breast cancer in 1969. After her loss, my father, who was a Presbyterian minister by training, spent much of his life researching and developing an immunotherapy to cure the disease that took his young wife. An autodidact with a ravenous intellect, a formidable power of recall, and access to the University of Colorado Medical

School library, he immersed himself in cancer research for over two decades, developing a working protocol which, with the support of outside investors, tested successfully on mice, dogs, and horses. A few years after his lead investor died suddenly of an aneurysm and funding dried up, he decided to share his research with no expectation of benefitting from it: In 2005, he published his work in *The Journal of Immune Based Therapies and Vaccines*. A decade later, when cancer came for him, it was like Beowulf perishing in a final confrontation with Grendel's mother, his intractable nemesis. If Beowulf had a pacifist son with no pretensions to be a warrior and no axe to grind against the Grendel family, that would have been me. I stumbled into this epic conflict without an agenda, focused only on getting through it with minimal damage.

I was the youngest of five children, and my mother first detected a lump in her breast around the time she became pregnant with me. As the pregnancy progressed, her breasts grew larger and she no longer felt the suspicious lump. When the cancer was diagnosed shortly after I was born, it turned out to be an aggressive form, requiring a mastectomy and a long, painful recovery. The cancer went into remission for several years but re-emerged as a throbbing pain in her legs, indicating the cancer had spread throughout her body. This time it roared back with a vengeance, and shortly before I turned 8, she died in bed at our home in Denver, Colorado. My memories of her are of a lovely, gaunt, dark-haired woman with tired eyes and infinite gentleness. She spent her waning days in bed and would occasionally invite me to sit and read *Winnie the Pooh* to her. She wore nightgowns of pale blue or yellow. There was always a heating pad nearby to ease the pain in her legs. The air in her bedroom was warm and close and smelled of Mentholatum ointment, a tin canister of which was never far from her bedside. In my darkest ruminations and my bleakest poetry, I have speculated on her state of mind as cancer closed in on her. In my own experience, I have seen only glimpses of the profound exhaustion and despair that cancer visits on its victims. I have come to believe that when her time arrived, my mother surrendered willingly, exhausted, wrung out from pain, welcoming death's oblivion, but hoping still for a Heaven.

At the time of my mother's death, her children ranged in ages from 17 to 7. My two sisters, both teenagers at the time, were probably affected the most, being robbed of their mother and role model at a vulnerable age. My brother Geoff and I were the youngest and always felt like we dodged some of the worst emotional damage. Years later, though, psychotherapy revealed to me I was mistaken. I simply sustained a different kind of damage, more elemental, like axe wounds that scar not a tree's bark but its very roots, and are manifest in every new branch and leaf it grows. As a family, we had to re-group, mourn, and move on collectively and individually. My brother David, the oldest, was a senior in high school, and in the fall of 1969 would start college at Northwestern University in Chicago. He was forced to deal with his grief as a sensitive young man settling in to an intense new social and intellectual world. Fifty years after my mother's death, David confessed he had a near-emotional meltdown after his freshman year as the grief he'd fled overtook him. Kristin, the second oldest, attended a high school where the turbulence of experimental busing made for a hostile, unsettled environment. Already traumatized by the death of our mother, she would go on to suffer another terrible loss soon afterward: Her boyfriend was killed by a drunk driver as he drove home from work. I remember hearing my sister wailing in her basement bedroom like a wounded animal. It was horrible even to consider so much grief in someone so young. My sister Cydney was in elementary school at the time. Willowy and dark-haired like our mother, she was surprisingly tough, or at least appeared to be, and periodically got in trouble for fighting in the hallways or mouthing off to a teacher. My father loved her spirit and couldn't hide his amusement when Cyd, having moved on to junior high school, called her prattling Latin teacher an asshole. Geoff and I were in elementary school when our mother died—he in fourth grade, I in second. We played football on the parkway in front of our house, wandered around the neighborhood with our respective groups of friends, and stumbled forward, mostly cheerfully, into adolescence, largely unaware of how much grief we carried with us.

The backdrop to all our lives, before my mother's death and after, was cancer. It lived with our family for years, wasting our mother away and depriving us all of a normal existence. When we came home from school, cancer was in the bedroom at the top of the stairs. And long after my exhausted mother slipped into a coma and exhaled her last breath, cancer hovered over our family like a suffocating fog. In his grief, my father raged against the God whose worship he led every Sunday—the God who, inexplicably, robbed him of his wife, and his children of their mother. Eventually he began to date a little; then he plunged precipitously into an ill-fated marriage with, it turned out, a mentally ill woman with four children of her own. Thus ensued a disastrous year of screaming matches, thrown objects, an overcrowded house, and occasional physical and emotional abuse by our stepmother. The sordid episodes ended after our stepmother, in a fit of rage, poured hot coffee over my father at the dining table. Their separation and divorce proceeded quickly after that, leaving our family with grim new wounds to heal.

Eventually my father married again; and this time he found a partner with whom he could spend the rest of his life: a tall, athletic, Denver native named Nancy Vandemoer. He and Nancy set about forging a durable and loving relationship while attending to the ragged state of affairs in our family. Shortly after they married, my father left his church, Montview Presbyterian, to focus on writing novels and researching his immunotherapy protocol. From then on, there were always oncology and immunology books and academic journals stacked neatly by his favorite reading chair in the living room, each meticulously underlined and annotated in red pencil. As his theory crystallized, he would share his work with us over the cocktail hour or at the dinner table. We comprehended few of his references to killer T-cells, GIK-therapy, and exogenous drug delivery. Mostly we sat and listened. It was an extraordinary experience: He spoke with the sophistication of an immunology PhD but in the inspirational tones of a practiced clergyman. Those of us who couldn't understand the science, I being chief among them, were swept along by his passion and the power of his language.

My father was always a crusader. As a young minister he

wasn't content to fulminate from the pulpit. He took the fight to the streets where, in Elizabeth, New Jersey, he organized against so-called "slumlords" who rented substandard housing to the poor. After he moved to New Rochelle, New York, in 1961 to be senior pastor at the North Avenue Presbyterian Church, he formed a citizens' task force against organized crime and its illegal gambling operation. His work quickly got the attention of the national press: *Look* magazine published a full-length feature on him and the group of courageous women with whom he worked, known as the "Irregulars." My Dad went on to write a book about this period of his life titled *The North Avenue Irregulars*, published in 1968. Shortly after the book appeared, Walt Disney purchased the movie rights and in 1979 released a comedy, only loosely based on the original, by the same title. I later learned that my father used the proceeds from the movie sale to pay off debt he incurred from my mother's medical expenses. After we moved to Denver in 1968, my father briefly re-engaged with his work against the Mafia, writing a report on the prevalence of organized crime in the Denver metropolitan area. But when my mother died in February 1969, he found a new crusade that would preoccupy him until the day he died.

In his haunting poem "The Convergence of the Twain," Thomas Hardy writes of the *Titanic*'s preordained collision with the iceberg that sank it that "No mortal eye could see/The intimate welding of their later history." Though my own convergence with cancer was far from epic, it felt just as preordained to me. When I consider the two strata of consciousness operating within me, I understood that my confident, optimistic self was always undermined by a doubtful self where existed a dim conviction that cancer and I must eventually meet. In that sense, I suppose, I had already been altered by cancer when I was a child growing up in a household hushed by worry. My mother's death ensured that cancer's imprint was deep and lasting. And my father's long, losing battle with the disease, first fought through research and then on his deathbed, exposed me to a broad spectrum of emotional and intellectual experiences with cancer. At one point, I told my wife that, when my cancer arrived on December 22nd, I wondered, *What took you so long?*

After my father married Nancy, a new level of calm descended on our home in the Park Hill neighborhood of Denver. Over the next few years, rooms were painted, new carpet installed, draperies upgraded, and furniture replaced. We began to feel like a normal household with a father, a mother, an old orange tabby named Chammy, and Duffy the dog. I moved on from Phillips Elementary School to Smiley Junior High School. But while the rest of my life was regaining some sense of calm, my time at school was tense. Racial tensions ran high, as they did everywhere in the "integrated" Denver Public Schools system. Smiley, and to a lesser extent, Manual High School, which I attended from 1976 to 1979, felt like a scene from *Lord of the Flies*, with lines drawn along racial divides and kids at violent odds with each other for no apparent reason. I was an introvert by nature and, except for a small group of close friends, kept pretty much to myself. After school we played basketball in the alley and football on the parkway. When skateboards came into vogue in the early '70s, I took up cruising around the neighborhood with my friends, looking for new asphalt on which to try 180s. When I was in sixth grade, my father gave me a white, five-speed stingray bike that I'd ride on summer evenings until sweat plastered my hair to my forehead. In my bedroom, I read *Lord of the Rings* and James Herriot books, and tapped out stories and poems on a futuristic white Olivetti typewriter. Fascinated by Middle Earth, I wrote my own fantasy novel based on troll dolls I'd played with as a child, all of them with names sounding straight out of Tolkien.

In high school I became more social, had a couple of girlfriends, and played, ever so briefly, on the lacrosse team. My grades were solid, though not up to the expectations of my father who believed I had intellectual gifts beyond what my grade point average indicated. When the time came, he encouraged me to apply to top colleges but recommended I include his alma mater, DePauw University in Greencastle, Indiana, as my safety. It's a good thing I did. Princeton, Amherst, Pomona, and William and Mary all sent me the dreaded thin envelopes expressing profound regret they could not offer me admittance. DePauw, on the other hand, welcomed me with a modest scholarship, making my decision uncomplicated, if a little disappointing. In August 1979, my parents put me on an airplane to Indianapolis, Indiana, and I was launched.

At DePauw I chose an English Composition major and Classics minor. Having written all my life and lived in a household where my father and oldest brother were published authors, I was inspired to become a legitimate writer. In 1983 I graduated *cum laude* and spent the following summer attending Middlebury College's Bread Loaf School of English at Lincoln College, Oxford. It was shortly after my plane landed at Gatwick airport in London that I met Barbara on the train platform there. We were attending the same summer program. We shared a train ride to Oxford together and, after an awkward first meeting, eventually started dating. If I was the underachieving English composition major from a so-so midwestern liberal arts college, Barbara was an East Coast intellectual thoroughbred. She was a tall, blue-eyed, preternaturally self-assured junior at Bryn Mawr College, an all-women's institution on an entirely different academic level from DePauw. There, she majored in English Literature and studied German and Philosophy with a seriousness that intimidated me. At Oxford, I studied Wordsworth and Coleridge; she studied Chaucer. I wrapped up my reading each night as quickly as possible so I could hit the pubs where we drank pints of Young's bitter and smoked Player's cigarettes. Barbara often declined to join us or showed up later, choosing instead to pore over her five-inch-thick volume of *Canterbury Tales* until she had mastered the assignment.

After Barbara graduated from Bryn Mawr, we coordinated our graduate school applications. I scrapped my initial plans to earn an MFA, opting instead to pursue a literature degree. Barbara had researched all the best graduate programs in English Literature, with Yale and the University of Virginia topping the list. We each developed our own list of prospective graduate schools but ensured that we had some overlap. I was accepted to UVa and Columbia. Barbara was accepted to UVa and University of Pennsylvania. Both schools offered her fabulous full-ride scholarships with generous stipends. My two schools offered me, well, admittance. We agreed on UVa, moved into a modest apartment on Brandon Avenue in Charlottesville, and began our studies. I finished my Masters Degree in 1986, opting not to continue for my PhD. Barbara, who came from a family of educators, had already committed to a career as an English professor: She continued on for her PhD, completing her dissertation in 1991 and receiving her degree that same year. Along the way, she won all kinds of accolades and became an attractive prospect to colleges looking for a new Victorianist.

While Barbara was wrapping up her coursework and writing her dissertation, I needed to earn some money. I tried various jobs, including a rideshare coordinator, a fitness instructor, and then a couple years as a stockbroker for A. G. Edwards and Sons. My time at Edwards proved two things to me: I had no talent as a salesman, and I possessed a terrible sense of timing. I received my Series 7 license—which authorized the bearer to sell securities like stocks, bonds, and mutual funds—in the spring of 1987, only six months before the stock market crashed on October 19. After that fateful day you couldn't give away stocks and bonds—or at least I couldn't—and my commissions dwindled pathetically. Within a year, I found a job more suited to my talents: running the custom publishing division of Charlottesville-based healthcare publisher, Kelly Communications. While at Kelly, I learned valuable lessons about business operations, leading teams, and pitching new accounts. By the time Kelly experienced fatal financial difficulties in the savings and loan crisis of the late '80s and early '90s, I had picked up enough skills to believe I could run a business of my own.

In 1991, Barbara went on the job market for a teaching position in nineteenth-century literature and received a number of offers, the best of which was at Skidmore College in Saratoga Springs, New York. We weren't yet married, and so had to decide what a move to Saratoga meant for our relationship. We decided it meant we'd get married that coming October. With Kelly Communications struggling to make payroll, I knew I'd either be looking for a job or starting my own business very soon, so I agreed to follow Barbara to Saratoga. She accepted the job at Skidmore, and I resigned from my Associate Publisher position. In the next few weeks I incorporated a new business, we moved to Saratoga, and Barbara started her new job. It was a blissfully turbulent time. We were too young to be scared of all we were taking on.

That was August 1991. We have lived in Saratoga ever since. Barbara went on to earn tenure and be promoted from assistant to associate and, eventually, to full professor. I built my fledgling content marketing business over the course of fifteen years, employing as many as fifty people at its peak, and then selling it in 2006 to a company based in Phoenix, Arizona. In 1998 our only child Madeleine was born, and suddenly we were a family. After selling my company, I chose to stay and help run the buyer's expanding East Coast operations. Our company went through two more mergers, growing into something big and unrecognizable, at which point I decided it was time to move on. In December 2015 I resigned and quickly formed a new LLC with a former colleague. Our plan was to purchase and merge three small marketing agencies with complementary capabilities, expand them through organic growth and subsequent acquisitions, and eventually sell to private equity or a strategic buyer, leaving behind a much larger, fully integrated marketing agency.

That formation of this new business turned out to be an important transition for me personally. I had spent the previous twenty-five years working feverishly to build some wealth and develop a professional reputation as a capable and principled leader in a not-so-principled industry. The plan to build a new business by combining smaller ones played perfectly to my skill set as an entrepreneur and strategist. My partner and I worked tenaciously for eighteen months to bring our vision to reality. During that time, we looked at over fifty small agencies, pitched private equity groups and mezzanine lenders for financing, and came within inches of closing a deal in the summer of 2017. That June, as we approached the finish line, one of the firms in our "roll-up" began to report shortfalls in its monthly earnings. Unable to reconcile its declining profits with the agreed-upon purchase price, we were forced to back away from the deal. It was a disappointing end to so many months of hard work, leaving my partner and me unexpectedly without a path forward.

One of the reasons I had left my previous firm was that I felt like a fish out of water there, both because the company culture had deteriorated badly, and because I started to sense a quiet but pervasive bias against older members of the leadership team. At 55, I was among the oldest people in the C-suite at a company populated largely by millennials, and recently taken over by a 40-something millennial wanna-be CEO. The marketing world, in particular, is obsessed with youth—young talent, young brands, young technologies. In that context, gray hairs don't garner the respect they otherwise might, for example, in a courtroom or on a board of directors. And though I had decades of hard-bought experience in building a successful firm, nurturing an inclusive work culture, buying and integrating businesses, and setting successful business strategies, I couldn't seem to overcome the fact of my age. Conspicuously, I didn't have a hipster beard and wear skinny jeans or talk rapturously about the latest social media app. I was feeling those first ominous sensations of forced obsolescence, and it pissed me off. There was no way I could stay; my pride as a professional demanded that I move on. By leaving my old firm behind and acquiring new businesses that needed senior leadership to continue their growth, I felt like I found the perfect use for my skills.

As my partner and I built our consultancy, I worked from home for a year and a half and, though I traveled extensively, I also got a feel for spending extended periods at home. When those periods weren't filled with work on our project, they felt disconcertingly like retirement. In those moments, and later when we wound down our business, I felt I was looking over a long, low river valley at the remainder of my life. It wasn't a view I had ever contemplated before—and I found the experience unnerving. It had never occurred to me that my giving notice in December 2015 might have been the terminus of my professional career. I never thought that the prestige, ambition, and accomplishment of being an entrepreneur and senior executive might be a thing of the past. Barbara was still working and was, by any measure, at the peak of her career. During that time she was finishing her third book; introducing dynamic new courses; sitting on committees; and organizing symposia. Her days were filled to capacity and she swept in and out of the house with all the purpose and zeal of a professional in overdrive. I was insanely proud of her accomplishments, and though I knew my career had up until then been an enviable and financially enriching one, I found myself longing for some of what she had. Just as much, I wanted to silence that voice in my head suggesting my time had passed, that my accumulated wisdom and insight had no place in the youth-obsessed culture of marketing.

After my partner and I closed up shop, I decided to enjoy the summer with my family. We went to Florence, Italy, where Barbara gave a paper at a conference. We then moved on to Paris and London, two of our favorite cities. Later that summer, when Barbara spent six weeks teaching at a graduate program in Tennessee, Mattie and I joined her for a week to enjoy the slow, southern pace and spend a weekend in Nashville checking out the honky-tonks and the Grand Ole Opry. In late August, we all went to Aspen, Colorado, where we share ownership in a house built by my stepmother's parents in the late 1940s. All that activity kept me busy and distracted, and silenced the voice in my head for a while. With the summer ending, I committed to doing some consulting gigs in the fall to keep my skills sharp.

While all this was happening, I was contending with another challenge that presented itself: In the summer of 2016, my daughter left for college. I always knew it would be difficult when Mattie left home, and Barbara and I would be transformed overnight into empty nesters. Having only one child meant that, for better or worse, Mattie got all our love and attention, and the three of us had grown tremendously close. My employment gave me the financial means to indulge my family in great experiences, and the flexibility to spend abundant time with Mattie as she grew up. We travelled to England, France, Italy, Costa Rica, Tanzania, and all over the United States. When Mattie took an interest in riding horses, we bought her a pony and, later, a Dutch Warmblood for show jumping. As Barbara and I found ourselves waiting at the barn for Mattie to finish riding lessons, I decided to take lessons as well. Before long, I owned my own horse and was spending summer weekends training at the barn and attending horse shows with my daughter. Our shared love of riding was the perfect way to bond; but, as I came to learn, it brought with it a pronounced sense of loss when she left for school at Barnard College. My only progeny had moved on, underscoring the fact that I was now the father of an adult; and my little girl and riding partner were gone as well.

Late that same summer, before Mattie was to leave for school, I drove out to the stable where we boarded our horses. It was a beautiful August day and, on any other such day, the two of us would have made that drive together, garbed in tan breeches and half-chaps. But that day, Mattie was at home packing for college and I needed to drop off some horse medications. As I approached the barn where we had spent countless summer mornings together, Mattie's absence took on a vivid, new reality and I found myself peering into what felt like a cold, black pit. Compounding the "loss" of my daughter was my own sense that I was moving from the relatively palatable space of middle age into something darker that I couldn't name yet. In that moment, Mattie's departure felt not like the beginning of a new phase in life, but like a sudden and terrible death of my identity as a father to a little girl, and the end of the richest, most satisfying time in my adult life.

As I walked through the barn that day, checking our horses and breathing in the smell of hay, Vetrolin, and saddle soap, the sense of despair I'd begun to feel on the drive overtook me. As if my body were responding to something more terrifying than my conscious self understood, my breathing grew rapid and shallow, my heart raced, and blood rushed in my ears. These were all sensations I'd encountered before in moments of fear or intense worry, but now they felt chaotic and unfettered, as if some restraint inside me had finally given out. As I placed the SmartPak supplement boxes in our tack trunks, I felt a cold sweat spread across my chest and back. Now completely rattled, I hurried back to the car where I sat with my hands on the steering wheel, trying to fend off the growing panic.

On the drive home I burst into tears.

At that point, of course, I had no knowledge of anxiety or panic attacks or the primitive fight-or-flight instinct that held me in its grip. I was simply terrified and had no idea why. Back at home, I busied myself with chores, avoiding Barbara and Mattie until I could collect myself. After an hour or so, the panic passed and I regained my composure. The next day it happened again, but was even worse.

Pretty quickly I realized I was experiencing some kind of anxiety and, knowing that things would only get worse as Mattie's departure date drew closer, I called my doctor. They had pills to get you through this sort of thing, after all. Dr. Quinn had cut back his hours in anticipation of retirement, so I met with his colleague, Dr. Amani. She listened to my account of what happened, gave me a once-over physically, and prescribed a thirty-day supply of Klonopin, an anti-anxiety medication. She also encouraged me to see a therapist to explore the emotional underpinnings of this new development.

One little yellow Klonopin pill later and I was nearly a new man. The anxiety subsided to a muted roar and I was able to get Mattie down to Barnard without too much emotional turmoil. Clearly that episode was a wake-up call and, out of curiosity as much as self-defense, I heeded Dr. Amani's recommendation to see a therapist. After a few unsuccessful calls to psychologists with no availability, I made a connection. Ranjit Bhagwat, a handsome young Chicagoan of Indian descent, returned my call, indicated he could take me on, and invited me in for a first consultation.

Since that time, I've enjoyed the remarkable process of excavating, with Ranjit's help, the oyster heap of emotions that is my mind. For the first several weeks, we dwelt on what it means to age, and to welcome a new phase of life without labeling the previous chapter as gone. We talked about identity and career, about being an adult male and feeling the cultural demands to earn money, perform gender-prescribed roles, and eschew displays of vulnerability. Ranjit listened and I talked. Some days I raged against this strange new place I had stumbled into. Other days I just wanted to talk about the book I was reading. Every now and then, Ranjit would stop me to dig deeper into something I said or to ask me to reframe my perspective slightly. The entire process was fascinating—and remains so. After having had so much resistance to therapy in the past, I now regret that it has such social stigma attached to it, at least for my generation. Millennials seem more comfortable texting their therapist's contact information to friends in need. I actually admire that openness. We could all benefit from therapy, I believe. I know I have.

So many forces converged at this midpoint of my life. I felt buffeted by powerful cross-currents: Looming physical decline, newly emergent anxiety, the apparent end of a long career and the professional identity I had constructed over twenty-five years, an entirely different relationship with my college-aged daughter, and the ringside seating at my wife's career triumphs. It all felt like plenty to handle at the time. In retrospect, therefore, I'm grateful I had about six months between winding down my LLC in June and the day I received my cancer diagnosis that December. Though I felt occasionally rudderless during that time, I was able to savor the emotional discoveries of my therapy, read broadly and enthusiastically, re-engage with creative writing, and enjoy having time with Barbara to redefine life without a daughter at home. But anxiety was never far away: Ranjit observed to me that, "Once your body realizes it can channel certain energies into a fight-or-flight response, it will always have that option." In other words, anxiety was here to stay, and medication was just a stop-gap measure for dealing with it. Therapy, and the tools and perspective it provided, was the prescription to help me tame the beast now living under my emotional bed.

My reading turned out to be an extraordinary balm at this bizarre new stage of my life—before the diagnosis and especially after. Having studied literature in graduate school, I had built up a good foundation of texts whose wisdom enriched and informed my life: Augustine, Boethius, Aquinas, Virgil, Homer, Wordsworth, Austen, Blake, Hopkins, Eliot, and Dickens. However, as my career had intensified and reading moved to the Internet and mobile devices, I read less literature and more CNN and ESPN on my iPhone. Reading had stopped being meaningful to me, becoming little more than the momentary absorption of headlines. I came to associate perusing online news with the rapid, shallow breathing of a panic attack—it feels like breathing, but it doesn't give the body what it needs. I longed to re-immerse myself in substantive texts and extract some wisdom with which to navigate this tractless wilderness my life had become. Before the cancer diagnosis I had started reading deeply about race, a subject of immense significance to me when I attended school in Denver. Why, I often wondered, did no one get along at school? Weren't we all too young to have ingrained racial hostility? Writers like James Baldwin, Eddie Glaude, Jr., Ta-Nehisi Coates, and Toni Morrison threw my intellectual windows open in a way no one ever had before. They led me to W. E. B. DuBois and to Manning Marable's biography of Malcolm X. As a break from race, I read about American history, soaking up Stephen Ambrose on World War II, and David McCullough and Richard Ketchum on the Revolutionary War. I returned to antiquity, reading Mary Beard's magisterial *SPQR* about the extraordinary expansion and administration of the Roman Empire. On particularly dark days after my surgery, I looked for spiritual comfort by picking up my mother's copy of Kahlil Gibran's *The Prophet* and even *The Oxford Annotated Bible*, which my father had given me. I'm not religious at all, but reading the New Testament brought back my Dad more vividly than any other means available to me. In the Gospel of Matthew, I heard my clergyman father's voice in every word and, consulting the Greek original in his seminary copy of the *Novum Testamentum Graece*, I came across his notes about upcoming exams on verb declensions. During that unsettled time, reading was, in a very real sense, my salvation.

Of course, once I was diagnosed and gained a more complete picture of my cancer, how far it had advanced, and what my treatment and recovery looked like, I began to spend a lot of time reading about prostate cancer. Understanding one's cancer means coming to terms with certain data points and statistics associated with your particular disease. The Internet is a rich resource for educating oneself on such matters; and I read a great deal about the prognosis for men with cancers like mine. The three numbers Dr. Z gave me after my diagnosis—my clinical stage, Gleason score, and preoperative PSA—became a kind of identity for me. Those data points tyrannized my thoughts for months; as some of them changed, not for the better, they became as important to me as my name and my age.

4

NAME, RANK, AND SERIAL NUMBER

THE DAY I received my diagnosis, Barbara and I persevered in our plans to go Christmas shopping for a few hours at an Albany mall. Our moods were predictably subdued but we were encouraged that my cancer seemed relatively manageable. It was also a relief not to be in diagnostic no-man's land any longer, to know what we were facing and have some concrete next steps. From Dr. Z's office we drove the short distance to Colonie Center Mall where we planned to while away the day buying Christmas stocking presents for Mattie, and last-minute gifts for siblings. There was a lot of snow and ice on the ground, so earlier that morning before I left for the doctor's office, I retrieved my hiking boots from the basement to keep my feet warm and dry for my stare-down with the Fates. After hurriedly lacing the boots on, I stood up and noted that the heels felt strangely spongy, something I hadn't recalled from previous seasons. No matter—they were comfortable enough and I was distracted by weightier issues. Later, when we parked the car at Colonie Center and began walking toward the mall entrance, however, I felt something flapping under my foot. Leaning against a car in the parking lot, I inspected my boots and found that the soles of both had deteriorated from months of damp storage and were peeling off at the heel. They were so rotten, in fact, that every step brought me closer to total shoe-failure and left black crumbs of pulverized rubber on the icy asphalt. By the time we stepped inside the shopping center, walking had become a challenge: Each time I raised a foot, seven inches of black rubber separated from the boot and, before the foot hit the ground, slapped back into place with a thwack. Inside that quiet mall, every flapping step was an embarrassment, announcing to the holiday shoppers of Albany, I mused, *the arrival of the village idiot.*

Watching me pick my way along the mall corridor, Barbara had trouble controlling her laughter. Under normal circumstances I would have had a good laugh with her. But today I didn't see the humor. Perhaps the fear and indignation of the last few days had caught up with me. Maybe I had low blood sugar or needed another cup of coffee. Whatever the reason, in that moment, I saw myself as a ridiculous figure, like Eliot's "Gerontion" grumbling, "Here I am, an old man." Only a few days earlier, I had been in the fetal position on an examination table with a biopsy probe in my rear. As of that morning, I had been handed a cancer diagnosis and faced treatment that can leave men incontinent and impotent. I was only 56, for Christ's sake. Now, just to make sure I felt the full force of my decrepitude, my shoes were disintegrating under my feet, giving me the absurd gait of a blue heron stalking crayfish in a swamp. We were not, as Queen Victoria once drily remarked, amused.

As luck would have it, there was an L. L. Bean store at the mall, and Barbara wisely suggested we make it our first stop. The store was warm and cheerfully lighted and, though it was fairly early on a Friday morning, dozens of shoppers milled around inside looking at parkas, flannel shirts, and day packs. Michael Bublé was crooning "Santa Baby" on the sound system. We quickly found the shoe section and, after a few minutes of comparing styles, I had swapped out my defunct footwear for a new pair of fleece-lined snow boots. On the way out of the store, I stopped at the customer service desk and handed my old boots to a pleasant looking older man with wire-framed glasses. "Can you throw these away for me, please?"

The man smiled and took the boots with their crumbling heels. "Well, I hope you bought a new pair. It's awful cold to go barefoot."

My mood improved, I mustered a perfunctory chuckle. It was a small thing to buy a new pair of boots, but it cheered me up. It was a problem we could fix—and sometimes you need a small win.

After we shopped a few more stores, we had lunch at a P. F. Chang's attached to the mall. We both ordered a beer with our meals, which was slightly out of character but somehow felt called for. Above our booth, dozens of amber lanterns hung from the ceiling. On the wall behind Barbara was a huge mural depicting elaborately robed Chinese men standing beside stout, short-legged horses. Picking at broccoli chicken and spring rolls, we talked about the diagnosis, Dr. Z's recommendations for an MRI, when and how we should tell Mattie, and a host of other issues. Most of all, though, Barbara was eager to understand the three statistics the nurse had written down. I shared what the doctor told me, which struck me as woefully limited—at least my memory of it was. It was clear to us both that these three numbers, recorded so emphatically in neat black ink on a sheet of paper, represented a new, complex, and pressing reality. It went without saying that each of us would be spending a lot of time on the Internet trying to understand their near-mystical importance.

Gleason score.

PSA.

Clinical stage.

These numbers and others—which can be updated or clarified along the way in your cancer treatment—become central to your identity as a patient: Men who have prostate cancer share them with each other like baseball cards at a swap meet. Several times, I came across cancer blogs on which every man, after posting a question or encouraging comment, signed off with his name, Gleason, and PSA number. It was the cancer version of name, rank, and serial number. Using just a couple of data points, you could discern so much about the man behind them: his prospects for recovery, how worried he and his family probably were, and the course of treatment he was likely considering. Like hieratic religious passages recorded on papyrus, these figures were a man's abridged narrative, the core essence of his cancer saga.

Based on my biopsy report, it appeared we had caught my cancer early. Only two of the twelve cores taken from my prostate showed malignancy and, of those, only 15 percent of each sample was cancerous. This suggested a small tumor. Additionally, my Gleason was a 6, which was also very encouraging. This score, I learned, is enormously important in gauging the risk presented by prostate cancer. The Gleason score was developed by pathologist Donald Gleason in the 1960s. In studying tissue samples from cancerous prostates, Gleason recognized that prostate cells go through distinct patterns as they mutate from normal cells to tumor cells. He scored cells on a scale of 1 to 5, with those closest to 1 being "low-grade" tumor cells that look and behave much like normal cells. Those at the higher end of the range are considered "high-grade," having mutated so much they look nothing like normal cells. These are more aggressive and likely to spread outside the prostate to other parts of the body.

Gleason grades are presented as the sum of two numbers, the first being the most prevalent type of cell present; the second number being the second most prevalent type. For example, a Gleason score of 6 would typically be presented as $3 + 3 = 6$. In the book Dr. Z gave me, it presents the Gleason "histologic grades" in a line-drawing illustration, with the low-grade cells appearing uniformly round and tidy. As you get to 3, they start to look more ragged, oblong, and disorganized. Gleason 4 and 5 cells look nasty—not like cells at all but like bits of torn paper. A Gleason score equal to or less than 6 is a low-grade tumor with excellent prospects for a full recovery. And though a $3 + 4 = 7$ is more aggressive, the prevalent cells are 3, which is still encouraging. This is what some doctors call a "good 7." It generally represents an intermediate risk. Then there is the $4 + 3 = 7$, which is scarier than the good 7. The most prevalent cells are more mutated and present a greater risk of spreading. This 7 I heard described as a "high-intermediate risk." When you get into high-risk Gleason scores of 8 and above, things get pretty concerning, with probability of metastasis or recurrence markedly higher.

As I mentioned, one's Gleason score may be updated in the course of diagnosis and treatment if new information is gathered. For example, two pathologists looking at the same biopsy samples might assign different Gleason scores. This actually happened to me when Sloan Kettering asked for and reviewed my biopsy samples from Dr. Z's pathologist, which I'll go into later. Additionally, if you undergo a prostatectomy, the surgically removed gland is sent to pathology for examination, at which point the pathologist assigns a more definitive Gleason score based on a comprehensive assessment of your malignancy. That Gleason number is the last, most definitive score you'll receive and matters a great deal in your prognosis.

In addition to my initial Gleason score, Dr. Z's nurse also wrote down my clinical stage of T1c. Now, staging a cancer has its own language and structure. To be honest, I didn't understand staging until I did a lot of research online. My confusion may have been due to some initial ambiguities in my cancer that made staging difficult—specifically, that my biopsy results suggested a small, relatively tame malignancy but that my PSA was high and getting higher. My PSA indicated that my Gleason score and clinical stage might not be corroborated by an MRI or post-surgical pathology report. My prostate cancer book laconically observed that a clinical stage of T1c means "prostate cancer is identified by needle biopsy for an increased PSA." Hell, I could have told you that. Still, on the long, vertical chart of clinical stages—ranging from T1 down to T4 (where the cancer has invaded "adjacent structures), to N (invasion of lymph nodes), to M (presence of metastases)—my cancer showed up reassuringly high on the list.

Like a Gleason score, the clinical stage may be updated as new information becomes available. If the MRI indicates your cancer has spread beyond the prostatic capsule (the thin skin on the outside of your prostate), or has invaded certain structures nearby, or has metastasized to the bones or distant organs, your clinical stage changes markedly. And, as with the Gleason score, once the surgeon has looked inside you, he or she can assess whether the biopsy or MRI presents the whole picture or if the cancer changed since then. In anticipation of receiving my surgical pathology, I become obsessed with phrases like "involvement" of "seminal vesicles," "lymph nodes," or the "bladder neck." I wanted to read that my "surgical margins" were clear, indicating the cancer had not spread beyond where the surgeon cut to remove tissue. Bad news on any of those items can change your clinical stage very quickly as well. I'll talk more in detail about my experiences with pathology reports later. But suffice to say, their significance can't be overstated.

I've referred multiple times to the immense significance of one's PSA score, which roughly correlates with the size and aggressiveness of your malignancy. My PSA score, we knew, was high and had velocity (meaning, it was increasing pretty fast), having moved from 15.4 to 19.6 in a few weeks. That was the part nobody liked and which led to the recommendation for an MRI. The postoperative PSA becomes a big issue as well: After your prostate is removed and your body has six or so weeks to flush any remaining antigen from its system, you are re-checked. At Sloan Kettering they look for a postoperative PSA of <0.05 ng/ml, which is essentially "undetectable." So precise is Sloan Kettering's red line on acceptable PSA levels that the mere absence of the "less than" symbol can be the difference between good news and bad. Assuming your PSA is in the undetectable zone, from that point forward, the patient is checked regularly, typically every three to six months, to ensure the PSA doesn't creep back up over time, which would indicate the continued presence of malignant cells. In such a case, a new discussion ensues on additional treatment options.

As I received these various prostate cancer statistics, or saw them updated, I was frequently surprised by how impenetrable, unreliable, even mutable such information can seem to the patient. This may be partly due to the fraught context in which such data is transmitted from doctor to patient. In the moments when I received my PSA score or pathology report, I was typically too distressed to fully understand what I was hearing. To some extent, I was able to mitigate this by inviting Barbara to my appointments so she could take notes and ask questions while I stared at my shoes, contemplating mortality and feeling my heart banging in my chest. The day I received my diagnosis, I was still hoping for a hall pass to a cancer-free future, so I hadn't done any preparatory reading on things like

Gleason scores and clinical staging; doing so would have struck me as unnecessarily defeatist. So when Dr. Z launched into a discussion about those very subjects, I simply wasn't prepared to understand them or to ask penetrating follow-up questions. When I did clear my mind and undertake some reading on my disease, I encountered alternative and even conflicting views on key points like PSA and Gleason numbers and what they portend. So much has been published on these subjects—survival rates for men with various preoperative PSA levels, the relationship of Gleason scores to recurrence, for instance—that the newly diagnosed patient can quickly become overwhelmed by all the nuances of research studies and the data they present in endless tables and charts. In this sense, both the emotionally charged context in which I received diagnostic information and the shifting landscape of research data made every statistic and every marker seem debatable, even subjective—much more so than is really the case, I think.

   That seeming mutability or inconsistency in interpretation, I surmised, underlies why Dr. Gleason in the 1960s had come up with a uniform approach to grading cancer cells. It's much easier to agree that the cells in question are a 3 or a 4 as opposed to "pretty good" or "totally fucked up." Those efforts at standardization are everywhere in health. The 1-to-10 scale for pain, as I mentioned in my introduction, is ubiquitous in examination rooms, with its illustrations of a smiley face at 1 and a grimacing face at 10. The same scale is used for the quality of erections at the Sexual Health Clinic and, I imagine, a host of other assessable phenomena. Even the language employed in pathology reports is rigorously defined for standard usage. The caption at the bottom of Sloan Kettering's reports reads:

   The following terms are used in MSKCC Radiology reports (except those of breast imaging studies) to convey the radiologist's level of certainty for a given interpretation.

   Consistent with > 90%
   Suspicious for/Probable/Probably approx 75%

Possible/Possibly approx 50%
Less likely approx 25%
Unlikely < 10%

These attempts at standardization struck me as a good thing, removing some of the ambiguity and contradiction inherent in human perspective and communication. But not all of it.

I mention all this because when you're in the thick of things with cancer treatment, sitting in the office of a urologist after a big test or procedure, the data starts to flow in a big way— typically when you are least able to consider it thoughtfully. As if that didn't confuse matters enough, for all the admirable efforts to standardize the terms used in diagnosis and treatment, surgeons and pathologists are still human beings with different interpretations, skills, biases, and perspectives. You won't always get the same assessment on some very important subjects. For that reason, it's enormously important to have someone with you whenever possible, even if you don't think you need it. In my earliest appointments before I knew I had cancer, I didn't include Barbara, either because I was trying to spare her the anxiety or simply didn't believe I needed someone else present. Not including her ultimately short-changed us both when it came to achieving clarity on key information. When Barbara was present, she was heroic—pressing the nurse or doctor for more detail, calling out contradictions, and acting as my advocate when I was feeling too banged up to speak for myself.

As difficult as it was to understand some of the initial information, I found it useful to regroup a day or two later to read up on what I'd learned. Of course, I would come across slightly different terminology or statements. One resource said you almost never see a Gleason score below 6 on a pathology report (in fact, since 2005, Gleason scores below 6 are rare). Other sources contradicted that. It didn't matter much. Anything at 6 or below is considered low-risk. But still, the sheer profusion of information made my research actually harder at times. For me, the way to overcome that confusion was to pick a few resources I respected (Sloan Kettering has fantastic content on their site, for example, as do other large non-profit cancer centers and teaching institutions) and stick with them for consistency of perspective. Wandering all over the Internet, where information ranges from invaluable to downright wrong, can actually be counterproductive. Plus, there's no substitute for talking with your doctor, asking probing questions, and pushing for more information. One of the key factors in how I chose a surgeon was how willing he or she was to sit and talk with me—without nervously glancing at the clock every few minutes. I had every right to understand all the information about my disease. Any good doctor should support that desire.

After our lunch at P. F. Chang's, Barbara and I did some more Christmas shopping, the normalcy of which rejuvenated us both, to some extent. Around 5 PM we drove to the Albany-Rensselaer Amtrak station to pick up Mattie, who had taken the Empire Service from Penn Station right after she wrapped up her final exams. When we spotted her coming off the escalator, she was still wearing "finals clothing"—sweats, an orange parka, and a baseball hat. Reed-thin and standing at five-foot-nine inches with blonde hair and blue-grey eyes, Mattie is a striking figure in any setting. We certainly had no trouble spotting her in a crowd of business commuters. If her height didn't give her away, her distinctive gait did: Mattie walks with a pronounced "turnout," often being mistaken for a ballerina, though she never took to dance. As she approached, lugging an over-full backpack on her shoulder and pulling a roller-bag behind her, she smiled as if to say, "You have no idea how tired I am." Knowing my workhorse daughter, I figured she was wrapping up a week of all-nighters fueled by matcha lattes and coffee. When I went to hug her, she didn't hug me back so much as present herself for my embrace, leaning into me with the weariness of a marathon runner at the finish line. With our only child returned home and in my arms, I allowed myself a moment to savor the smell of her hair, the sweetness of a college semester completed, and Christmas vacation stretching before us. This holiday would not be without its complications, of course, but it was still worth drinking in.

On the drive home it snowed heavily. Not wanting to cook dinner when we got back to Saratoga, we picked up some takeout from a Moroccan restaurant in Troy, only fifteen minutes from the train station. At home, we ate our dinner, heard all about Mattie's final exams, watched a little *Shark Tank*, and collapsed into bed early.

We hadn't decided when or how to tell Mattie about my cancer diagnosis. That was for another day.

5

DISCLOSURES

THE MORNING AFTER MATTIE came home, we mustered the courage to tell her about my diagnosis. That was a Saturday just two days before Christmas, and the timing was unfortunate, but we felt strongly she needed to know and we didn't anticipate a better opportunity to break the news. The three of us sat down in the family room and I, with a hot cup of coffee steaming on the table beside me, calmly told Mattie all about my diagnosis. I presented prostate cancer to her much as Dr. Amani had to me: It's the good cancer, something to take seriously but not get worked up over, fixable with surgery or radiation. She listened intently, then reached over and gently gripped my upper arm, saying softly, "Oh, Daddy boy." The whole disclosure went well. Seeing the expression on Mattie's face and hearing my own choice of words, I was reminded why we so often employ euphemism when speaking of cancer. While I came to resent how we paint prostate cancer with the rainbow and sparkles of optimism, I resorted to that exact representation to avoid worrying my daughter. In that, I suppose, I was a total hypocrite. But my motives were pure and, for better or worse, the language I used appeared to soothe her. While she seemed satisfied with our presentation of the risks, I suspect she was worrying a great deal more than she showed. I glimpsed her anxiety in the questions she asked and in how she studied my face as I talked—as though attempting to discern a deeper truth from my expressions. I finished by telling her that my MRI was scheduled for January 4th and that it would give us important new insight into my cancer.

Talking to Mattie, I found myself bitterly regretful that I had brought this worry into my family. Eventually, Ranjit heard me say something to this effect in a therapy session, and asked pointedly whether I had *asked* for this cancer. I readily comprehended his meaning but couldn't shake the feeling that I had burdened my family with an anxiety they didn't deserve. Even if it wasn't my fault, it angered me—much more than having cancer did. What father doesn't pride himself on being a bulwark against worry? Now I had become a source of worry for those I loved, and that made me feel only more vulnerable and imperfect. If leaving my job had dealt a blow to my sense of self as provider and protector, having cancer was driving the sword in deeper.

Once Mattie had been informed, I faced the decision of whom else to tell about my diagnosis. Because I was very close with my four siblings, there was no doubt I would tell them immediately. But the question remained whom else I would bring into the circle of trust. Barbara and I talked at length about this, neither one of us inclined to widen the circle for now. My general sense was that telling people so early in my cancer treatment would raise more questions than it answered—that I would only generate anxiety and speculation without being able to provide any resolution. I envisioned myself fielding constant phone calls, texts, and emails inquiring about the latest test results or appointment and, ironically, my having to play the role of communications liaison and chief consoler. Looking back, that concern was probably way over-blown; but at the time, I just didn't have the emotional energy to invest in sharing information. So we limited the disclosure of my diagnosis to Barbara's and my siblings. As I will discuss later, the decision of whom to inform, how much to disclose, and when became something of a mental exercise for me—and I seldom felt like I got it entirely right. One thing I know for certain, however, is that it's an intensely personal choice for the cancer patient. And, frankly, anyone who disagrees with when he is brought into the circle, or how much he is told, should keep that opinion resolutely and silently to himself.

With all those considerations bouncing around in my mind, I resolved to inform my siblings the same day I told Mattie, so I wrote them a group email. By doing so, I could reach them all at the same time, give them the same facts, and establish a precedent for communicating treatment updates in the future. After all, I had spent a career devising communications strategies for clients, and these issues mattered to me. I drafted a straightforward note that shared the major details of my journey so far and then asked Barbara to check it for clarity and tone. I didn't gloss things over as much with my siblings as I had with Mattie, but I did keep it upbeat. Geoff was the first to respond, calling within minutes of my sending the note. He was at lunch with his wife Margie but stepped away from the table when he received the email on his phone. Born only a year and a half apart, Geoff and I had been extraordinarily close since we were little boys. Because we were always together—playing football, running around the block, or wrestling in the basement—my father had the habit of asking other siblings simply, "Where are the boys?" Or "Someone tell the boys it's dinner time." As we became men with families and jobs, we consulted each other on major parenting or career decisions, almost always agreeing on the proper course of action. Geoffrey was proud, loyal, and principled in a noble, old-fashioned way. For him, there was no gray area in considerations of right and wrong; and when I was stymied by a matter of moral ambiguity, he seemed to see the answer immediately. Mostly, though, Geoff was fiercely committed to those he loved, willing to go to extraordinary lengths to provide support.

I shouldn't have been surprised, therefore, that Geoffrey was almost belligerent about my diagnosis. He grew up with the cancer storm cloud over his head, just as I did. But I don't believe Geoff saw an eventual meeting with cancer as inevitable; it was something to keep at bay by any means possible. My fatalism would have offended his sense that there is a discernible arc of justice to the universe. Geoff was like my father, inclined to pick up a sword and head for the battlefield, inflamed with righteous indignation. What made him angry in this case, though, was that I had the cancer and there was nothing he could do to help. "Buddy," he said, "I just can't believe you have to deal with this."

"I know, but it'll be fine. It looks like we caught it early."

He paused for a long time and I could hear the ruckus of the restaurant in the background. When he resumed talking, I could tell he was on the verge of tears. "You know if there's anything you need . . . ."

"I know that."

"You want me to fly up for your MRI?" he asked, almost begging for a way he could provide support.

I thanked him for the offer but asked him just to send lots of positive thoughts.

In the email to Geoff and my other siblings, I explained that my next big step was an MRI, so they all knew it was my primary focus. For Geoff, who so badly wanted to take some kind of action, the days of helpless anticipation leading up to my MRI would be particularly hard. I admired his earnestness more than he knew. Too often, I felt, my own empathy waned in the face of pragmatism or mere distraction. Geoffrey never let that happen. He was the guy who would write the date of my MRI in his calendar and call the day before to check in. The authenticity of his empathy made his expressions of concern just as genuine. At least in my experience, he never succumbed to platitudes or awkwardness when talking about emotionally charged issues, which made it easy to speak candidly with him about my cancer.

Over the course of that day, my other siblings all responded to the email. Their notes were lovely, thoughtful, sincere. Our family history with cancer ensured that each of them comprehended the tangled emotional context in which my email was written. They didn't need to say much to impart their subtle understanding. Reading their notes, I felt my family's support like a wind at my back. It was a good thing, too, because waiting for the result of that MRI was weighing heavily on my mind.

In one of my therapy sessions, I expressed to Ranjit my reluctance to tell people about my diagnosis. I told him how, when one of my former employees was diagnosed with aggressive breast cancer, I struggled with how to express my sympathy. Having felt that unease firsthand, I was certain others would feel it with me. I didn't fault them for it, but I also didn't want to deal with it. Ranjit, who counsels numerous cancer patients, observed that our culture hasn't yet found the right way to talk about the disease. "We're all so terrified of getting cancer," he said, "that our immediate instinct is to react with fear for ourselves."

That struck me as absolutely right.

"When you get cancer," he continued, "you become a reminder to people that *anyone* can get it at any time. It's just too random and scary for us to deal with."

I have no idea how to overcome that dynamic. There must be layer upon layer of social psychology to excavate there. Fundamentally, though, I think we need to demystify cancer at the interpersonal level—to work toward an open acknowledgement that, sure enough, everyone lives in fear of that diagnosis. If cancer reminds us all of our human vulnerability and that long shadow of mortality that haunts every one of us, then the diagnosis of a friend or loved one is an opportunity to share our fears and root each other on against a common enemy. Too often, though, our own unease makes that simple moment of bonding devolve into blather about thoughts and prayers. God knows, I've written my share of get-well cards with banalities like, "I know you'll beat this!" I always meant well, but I could have done so much better.

It's funny, I definitely got hung up on certain words and phrases people use in talking about cancer. One particular verb really made me bristle: *battle*. Early on, Barbara used that word occasionally, before we knew exactly what we were facing. I'm sure it was her way of girding up her own loins, so to speak, for what lay ahead. No doubt, when one feels assaulted, using assertive language to counter the assault is empowering; I respect that. I didn't take issue with the use of terms like "battle" or "struggle" *per se*; I just took issue with them being used about me. You have to remember that, until my surgery and recovery, I never suffered from any adverse effects of my cancer. Aside from the usual aches and pains of middle age, I felt like a healthy male specimen. I reserved the use of "battle" for people who were fighting for their lives against advanced cancers. We hear all the time about women who are "bravely battling breast cancer" or the man who died after a "valiant battle against pancreatic cancer . . . " I didn't see myself battling anything yet, and I certainly hoped never to start. The plan was to get treated with surgery or radiation, beat the shit out of prostate cancer, and then get back to living life. If we found later the cancer had spread and I needed additional treatments against a now-entrenched foe, okay, that's where the battle started; but I wanted no part of that.

No doubt, word choice mattered a lot to me and, I'm sure, to every cancer patient. We read meaning into everything. Did I get neurotic at times about it? Absolutely. But cancer can quickly make even the calmest person become an obsessive hypochondriac. It wasn't just word choice that affected me, either. I remember times when Barbara discussed my cancer in phone conversations with her siblings. Because she's so close to them all, she was frequently candid about her worry, at times crying gently when I wasn't in the room. Occasionally I would overhear these tearful exchanges and was surprised by how much they spooked me. Was I fooling myself about my prognosis? Did Barbara know something I didn't? I may have had that reaction because she and I had been so united in our experience of the disease that I was startled to hear an outlook on my cancer we hadn't formed together. That momentary divergence in our perspectives threatened the fragile hope I rallied every morning when I awoke, nurtured all day long, and took to bed at night. I needed to believe that, as the patient, I was the only person given to pessimism, so that anyone familiar with my diagnosis would immediately and objectively view my outlook as sunny. I already had all the fear and trembling I could handle.

Outside the circle of my family and closest friends, I generally observed one of two reactions when telling people about the diagnosis. Some responded with grave concern, asking if they could help or how I was feeling. Though I genuinely appreciated their concern, as with Barbara's conversations with her siblings, it unsettled me. It was only after I felt more optimistic about my prognosis that I could reassure these worried well-wishers that I was on the road to a complete recovery. Doing so allowed me to snatch confidence from the jaws of worry, so to speak. Others I told expressed relief that it was "only" prostate cancer. I'm sure they said this to reassure me. But as I wrote earlier, this response made me feel they were dismissing the whole thing— the "starter cancer" concept.

I also found that some people took it personally when I didn't tell them right away. One friend of mine was amazed I'd kept it "under my hat" for so long. "Hell, man, I would have called you right away to complain about it," he laughed. Others seemed to resent being told only after I was through with surgery, as if my sharing the information earlier would have conferred membership in an inner circle, but I might have felt the same way. The fact is, I told as few people as I could get away with, so I could focus more on dealing with my own worry and less on fielding inquiries from others. Perhaps that was selfish, I don't know.

As time passed, I grew more comfortable with my identity as a person with cancer and, when I was sufficiently reassured that the worst was behind me, began to share my story with a broader circle of friends and acquaintances. Those conversations generally took place after my six-week PSA test, which meant I could recount the narrative in an emphatic past tense. Most often, the opportunity to divulge the news arose over cocktails or dinner. As was generally the case in small social gatherings, the question "So how've you been?" eventually came around to me, and I'd take the opportunity to answer honestly. I felt a little sorry for people who asked. They showed the startled regret of hikers who stumble upon an agitated moose in a forest clearing. At that point, I imagined, they just wanted to backtrack. At least I could soften the whole thing by starting with the good news—the way you tell someone you had a car accident: "Everyone's fine but I just wrecked the Honda." Over time, I got better at putting people at ease as I told the story. Doing so involved a careful balance of candor and euphemism, objectivity and optimism. Almost without exception, the conversation would end with some version of, "I'm so sorry you had to go through that. But we're just glad it worked out okay." Mission accomplished for everyone concerned.

Communicating about cancer is a fraught subject any way

you decide to handle it. Those with the disease must decide whom to tell, when to tell them, how many details to provide, and what the implications are for sharing the news. Each time I told someone—and depending on his or her response—I felt either relief or regret. In my most cynical moments, I was tempted to critique people's responses. I remember in the movie *Something's Gotta Give* with Jack Nicholson and Diane Keaton, Harry remarks with exasperation to Erica, "Try not to rate my answer." I admonished myself in similar terms. It doesn't help matters, I realized, to assess who got it "right" and who didn't. Doing so only treats the disclosure of a cancer diagnosis like a mystery rite, and that's the last thing we need.

The same day I told Mattie about my diagnosis and sent an email to my loved ones, I set about researching treatment options. Though my ailment still felt entirely conceptual, I had a mounting desire to develop a game plan. I began the process by talking to two men who had already been treated for prostate cancer, my brother-in-law Frank and my close friend Terry. Frank was a malpractice lawyer who had done well for himself, living with my sister in a sprawling townhouse in Lone Tree, Colorado, a suburb of Denver. He was a sweet guy with a passion for history and single-batch whiskey, and, though he and my sister had married only a few years before, I had already developed a genuine fondness for him. He had been diagnosed about a year before me, and when I had received Kristin's email sharing the news, I took the view, as many people do, that prostate cancer wasn't a big deal and Frank would be up and at 'em in no time. I promptly sent him a note expressing my concern and kept an eye out for my sister's updates on his treatment—but I had no idea what he was really going through. From Kristin's periodic emails, I learned that Frank had opted for external beam radiation with radioactive seeds implanted in the prostate. I remember being impressed that such an option— or combination of options—even existed. It all sounded very space-aged and encouraging. I imagined my brother-in-law lying on a table in a gleaming medical laboratory, his cancer cells being vaporized by a beam of pulsing green light—all while bespectacled doctors nodded approvingly from behind a glass window. That's how removed I was from the reality of cancer—and that's how most people are.

Thus, from the moment I was diagnosed, I knew Frank would be one of my first conversations and, before I had a chance to reach out, he called me from his car on his way to work. As he spoke, I could hear the rush of traffic in the background. Now, as an attorney, Frank is a thorough researcher, which became more evident as we talked. If he was handling a lawsuit about glioblastoma treatment, he had to become a lay expert in that disease, and did so through exhaustive research. His expertise in prostate cancer was immediately obvious. He asked how I was coping with the worry, and then quickly inquired about my PSA and Gleason numbers. He listened carefully and said something like, "Well, with a Gleason of 6 and only two cores showing cancer, you're in good shape. That's very encouraging." He went on to mention that eight of his cores had shown cancer, indicating a much larger tumor than mine. Plus, he said, his Gleason was a "good 7," 3 + 4 = 7, which was slightly more advanced than my 6. He laughed that he "researched the shit out of prostate cancer," having gone so far as to speak with a couple of nationally famous specialists. As I listened, I was secretly hoping he could save me some work by sharing some of his notes.

He then turned to the subject of surgery versus radiation, explaining that he knew early in his research that he would never consider surgery. "If you start considering surgery as an option," he went so far to say, "call me and I'll talk you out of it."

I laughed.

"Seriously, Jimbo. When the doctor told me you have dry orgasms, I think that was the kicker."

"Whoa."

"I mean, what the fuck? Are you kidding me? And then there's the risk of impotence and even incontinence."

I was taking notes as he talked, stumbling over the spelling of *incontinence*.

When he heard that cure rates are the same for surgery and radiation, but that radiation has fewer of those risks, he added, it was a slam dunk. His voice got a little high-pitched as he talked.

I asked if he was happy with how things had turned out.

He said that he was, but that there had been "changes" to get used to—and that he went through six months of hormone therapy prior to radiation, which reduced his testosterone levels to zero. He did not love those six months, and he emphasized with obvious relief that it was behind him.

"No testosterone?" I gasped, suddenly trying to dismiss from my mind the image of Frank with budding breasts.

"It's not as bad as you think. I just spent a lot of extra time at the gym to maintain my muscle tone during that stretch."

We talked more about the radiation technology. Frank knew the facts with remarkable clarity and detail, but he lost me when he got into discussing protons and beams and seeds. My takeaway was that Frank was extremely pleased with his outcome and advised passionately against surgery. His zeal was persuasive: Radiation good. Surgery bad.

Frank's takeaway, he later confessed to me, was that my PSA was alarmingly high. Though his tone on the phone was nothing but encouraging, he admitted that when he'd hung up, he felt deeply concerned that there was more to my diagnostic picture than met the eye. Here, his expertise served him well.

Before we finished our conversation, I told him I read that if you select radiation as your primary treatment, your options are limited if the cancer recurs, with surgery being almost ruled out.

"Yeah, that's true. Radiation changes the tissue down there and makes surgery very tricky afterwards," he agreed.

"So what would you do if the cancer came back?"

"I'm not sure," he said after a pause. "Your body can take only so much radiation. But you know, if I live five fewer years with better quality of life, I'll take that. I couldn't live with the idea that I might end up in diapers, you know?"

Sensing it was time to change the subject, I moved on to some family news, and then we hung up.

Frank was the poster child for radiation therapy, I thought. And as passionate as he was about his choice, he was equally clear on the evils of surgery. His conviction and the impressive research he'd done invested him with tremendous credibility. I came away from the call pretty well convinced that radiation was the way to go. What hadn't occurred to me yet was that Frank and I had distinctly different circumstances, and mine were changing with every disclosure of diagnostic data I received.

My next conversation was with Terry, one of my closest friends who'd had prostate cancer about eight years earlier. Before he moved to North Carolina to retire with his wife Michele, he had been Barbara's and my fitness trainer in Saratoga. During the years we worked out together, Terry and I formed a deep and enduring friendship; so it felt strange that I knew so little about his experience with the disease. Frank and I were separated by a couple thousand miles, but when Terry was diagnosed and treated, he lived in Saratoga Springs and was, except for a brief break during his surgery and recovery, training with us.

We had first met Terry at a cocktail party at the home of a mutual friend. Being an introvert, I was sipping a scotch, hanging close to Barbara, and counting the minutes until we could go home. My party-loving wife, I could tell, was itching to circulate. Knowing I'd have to start socializing soon, I scanned the room for familiar faces. About twenty feet away from us, standing with a small group, was a tall African-American man with luminous chestnut skin; a broad, disarming smile; and a Questlove-style afro that took me right back to my high school years in Denver. A six-foot-two-inch black man with a '70s-style natural was not a common sight in white-bread Saratoga, so I was already intrigued. On top of that, he was dressed so stylishly that every other man in the room looked like a pair of wrinkled khakis by comparison. I remember Terry wearing a black velvet sport coat with a baby blue pocket square, jeans, and a pair of sleek suede loafers. I think of myself as having some sartorial sense, but Terry had a bold, pronounced personal style I hadn't encountered before, and I loved and envied him for it.

A few minutes after I spotted Terry in the crowd, our hosts appeared and guided us over to meet him and his wife Michele, an insurance executive at State Farm. When Barbara learned that Terry was a personal trainer, she asked for his business card, after which a long, surprisingly comfortable and boisterous conversation ensued, covering everything from weight training to 1970s funk to ballroom dancing (which Terry taught as well). The four of us have been like family ever since. When I would work out with Terry in his state-of-the-art home gym, he'd play ESPN on the television while I did mountain climbers or push-ups at his instruction. Between sets we'd talk about Floyd Mayweather's upcoming bout, or Eli Manning's latest playoff performance. We were both fans of African-American comedy, and Terry, who astonished me with his power of recall, would crack me up with his rendition of Richard Pryor's pet monkey routine. I swear, I pulled more muscles laughing with Terry than I did working out.

While I tend to be a little gloomy in my outlook, Terry made it a practice to be unfailingly optimistic. When I griped about politics, he would counter that politicians are just human beings trying to do their jobs under difficult circumstances. Anything I complained about, he found a silver lining. It was a remarkable discipline he had developed. So it was a clinic in optimism when he took me aside before my workout one day to tell me about his prostate cancer diagnosis. As he tended to be in all aspects of his life, Terry was extraordinarily precise in sharing the details of his diagnosis. I listened carefully, watching his face for indications he might be more worried than he let on. But he was a picture of inner peace. He explained that he and Michele were telling only a few close friends and that he would be laid up for a while after surgery and consequently wouldn't be able to train me for a few weeks.

I asked where he was receiving treatment.

"Right here in Saratoga, my brother," he responded with his usual warmth. "Michele and I like my urologist a great deal so we decided to have him perform the surgery." He went on to explain that his surgeon was trained in robot-assisted prostatectomies, using a technology called DaVinci. Evidently, this same surgeon had been recruited by Saratoga Hospital specifically for his expertise with DaVinci technology, and had been training other local surgeons in its use.

To hear Terry tell it, his surgery was going to be a breeze. He indicated they had discovered the cancer early, anticipated no difficulty in removing it, and expected a full recovery with no real concerns for his long-term health. When he told me all this with his trademark optimism, I think my brain scribbled somewhere on a notepad "Terry fine" and "prostate cancer manageable." As a result, on some subconscious level, I didn't engage as meaningfully with the reality that a close friend was facing cancer and undergoing major surgery that could have a long-term impact on his life. It was as if my impulse toward active empathy went limp when he flashed that reassuring smile. I'm not proud of my response. What's worse, it wasn't even a conscious one.

That's not to say I was disengaged. The fact is, we were pretty solicitous about Terry's surgery and recovery. We asked all about his progress and showed love at all the appropriate places, but I simply wasn't prepared to offer the kind of empathy Terry deserved. As he predicted, my friend sailed right through the whole thing—or appeared to—which made my passivity feel more excusable. Everything happened as he said it would, and within weeks he was doing his wild-eyed Muhammad Ali impression—"I shook up the world!"—between my sets of dumbbell rows. Though Terry turned out fine, I see the whole episode as a missed opportunity to deepen our friendship through empathy. Instead, what Terry got was the emotional version of a bro hug and a slap on the back. He deserved so much more than that.

In January 2018, when I called Terry to tell him about my own diagnosis, I tried to show the same optimism and spirit he'd displayed to me years before. I made some stupid remark about admiring him so much I decided to get prostate cancer, too. I don't think it struck the right tone, momentarily confusing Terry on whether I was telling a joke or breaking bad news. Nonetheless, he listened with a grave intensity that suggested perhaps his cancer experience hadn't been quite as sunny as it appeared. After hearing all about my random PSA test and subsequent diagnosis, he paused for several seconds, then began speaking in his rich baritone.

"First of all, J, thank God you caught it when you did. I mean, that could have been a nasty situation if it went undiagnosed."

I agreed that I had been very lucky.

"You're young and in great shape, so I have no doubt you'll cruise right through this." As he spoke, it occurred to me I was about Terry's age when he was diagnosed. That realization and his unfailing optimism buoyed my spirits. I asked him about his surgery and recovery. His experience, or at least how he told it, was nearly ideal: No complications from the surgery and minimal incontinence, with just a little "dribble" here and there after he urinated. He said he was back to normal functioning in a few months, but new and improved. He added, in fact, that before his surgery, urination had been a slow and halting affair due to his enlarged prostate, but now, well, he was a freaking racehorse. We laughed uproariously. Listening to Terry, I remembered *Love in the Time of Cholera* and Urbino's "stallion's stream . . . so potent, so replete with authority." I thought, too, of watching in astonishment as my Canadian Warmblood Kieffer, through the sheer force of his redolent urine, drilled a foamy hole deep in the shavings on the stall floor. How satisfying it must have been for Terry to regain his own stallion stream and feel like one aspect of advancing age could be rolled back. Surgery was starting to sound less and less like the worst-case scenario.

Because Terry and I kept very little from each other, I asked how things were working from a sexual perspective. He readily volunteered that he had taken Viagra for a few months after the surgery, but fairly soon didn't need it anymore. Listening to all this I thought, *I've got to see Terry's surgeon.* Just as my conversation with Frank convinced me radiation was the answer, Terry made surgery sound like a urologic equipment upgrade.

"Things really came together well for you, didn't they?" I said with a mix of admiration and relief.

"They did," he replied. "I feel pretty blessed, because it doesn't always go that well—especially for older guys who might have other health problems."

After I hung up with Terry, I was heartened by his results but had no real clarity on the surgery-versus-radiation dilemma. Consequently, I went back online to do more research on side effects. While looking at a prostate cancer blog, I came across a post that underscored Terry's final remark about age. The story, posted by JoeBiz49 (whose birth year I took to be 1949, putting him at 68 years old), detailed how he had undergone a prostatectomy for a low-risk malignancy with a Gleason 6. After his surgery, he experienced rampant incontinence, going through several pairs of diapers every day. As months passed, his incontinence barely improved, preventing him from golfing, dining out, or even taking long walks with his wife. Finally, a year after his surgery and fed up with having his life on hold, JoeBiz49 returned to his surgeon to have an artificial sphincter implanted to stanch his seemingly endless flow of urine. The post was a cautionary tale to those considering a prostatectomy, though he also acknowledged that the severity of his problems had statistically low odds—a fact that didn't really help him. It was a sobering narrative; and I couldn't help imagine the toll his incontinence had taken on his self-esteem, relationships, and expectation of living a fulfilling life after cancer. JoeBiz49's story was the photo negative of Terry's and reminded me that, just because Terry and Frank apparently sailed through treatment, not everyone does.

When my date with the MRI machine arrived on January 4th, I was having flashbacks to my previous encounter with the amazing donut-shaped machine. Back in 2005, I had developed an array of unsettling neurological symptoms, including nerve pain on the left side of my body and strange, electrical paresthesias all over, for which my neurologist ordered an MRI to rule out multiple sclerosis. Aside from being freaked out by the mere possibility I could have MS, I remember being fascinated by the machine: a giant, white cylinder, extending into the center of which is a platform on which the patient lies. Twelve years ago, when I was loaded into the machine to have my brain and spinal cord scanned, I lay there stock-still as a voice on an intercom gave me instructions: hold my breath, breathe, hold my breath again. I heard a whirring sound, and something inside the machine spun around me at terrific speed, all the while taking ghostly pictures of my central nervous system. A few days later I learned I didn't have MS and that the paresthesias were probably caused by a virus wreaking havoc on my sensory nerves. They couldn't say for sure. When my neurologist called to give me the MRI results, I had been having lunch with Barbara at an Italian restaurant, enjoying the May sunshine at an outdoor table. We toasted my good news with red wine and together breathed a sigh of relief. So, all things considered, I had reasonably positive associations with MRIs.

My prostate MRI in January proceeded pretty much the same way, except now they were scanning my groin—and I already knew my diagnosis. The current objective was more specific: to determine why my PSA was so high when the tumor, based on the pathology report, looked so small. Because these results could dramatically change my prognosis, as the day approached, I became increasingly tense. We might learn that the tumor was bigger than previously thought, had escaped the prostatic capsule, or even that it had spread to my lymph nodes or, God forbid, bones. It was a significant next step in my diagnosis and would likely guide my treatment choices. The procedure went as uneventfully as it had the time before, and before I left, I obtained a CD of the images so I could share the results with my second- and third-opinion doctors.

When Dr. Z ordered my MRI, he also scheduled for me to come in and review the results 10 days after the procedure. When I told him I didn't want to wait that long for the results, he recommended I call his office at any point forty-eight hours after the MRI and he would give me a preview. Accordingly, I let two days pass after the MRI and called his office right when they opened at 9 AM. Dr. Z was unavailable but the receptionist promised to leave him a message.

No return call came that day.

Slightly aggravated, I let another day go by and called again. Around 4 PM that day Dr. Z called me back. He was between patient appointments and sounded harassed. The MRI identified a larger tumor than was indicated by the biopsy, he explained. It was located on the left side of the prostate and out of the reach of the biopsy needle. He went on to share some technical-sounding dimensions and added that the tumor size helped answer why the PSA was so high. All this, he said, corroborated his theory about my PSA and tumor size. He was obviously pleased with his prognostication. I was a good deal less enthusiastic. Predictably, I had lots of questions but was having difficulty articulating them and, as I paused to gather my thoughts, Dr. Z said, "So we'll talk more about this when you come in. Believe it or not, I have patients waiting."

Believe it or not, I have patients waiting? I played the phrase back in my head a few times after I hung up to see if it sounded any better in reruns. In fact, it sounded worse.

I mentioned earlier that there are milestones in one's relationship with a doctor when trust is strengthened or damaged. This was the second milestone. The first was when Dr. Z opposed my having an MRI before my biopsy, but I had been willing to work past that disagreement. After all, in most other respects, he had been perfectly pleasant to deal with, if slightly lacking in bedside manner. But now I was hearing what sounded like sarcasm, and there was no legitimate reason for that. Up until that point, I had been committed to pursuing treatment in either Saratoga or Albany. But perhaps I hadn't been thinking far enough ahead, or maybe I assumed a major cancer center wouldn't be covered by insurance. It was more of a visceral position than a rational one, I think. Albany is no podunk town, so it would have been needlessly elitist, I felt, for me to ignore the treatment options in my own area. But all of that changed when Dr. Z, however unintentionally, belittled my interest in the MRI results. Of course, I always planned to obtain a second and third opinion on my course of treatment, so Dr. Z was never a foregone conclusion as the provider of choice. But now he was on the verge of being ruled out entirely.

As a matter of fact, before that unfortunate exchange with Dr. Z, I had begun researching alternative sources of care: I searched online for the nation's leading institutions for prostate cancer treatment; I talked to friends and family who had dealt with the disease. I also brought to this process some prior knowledge of the most respected medical organizations in the US. My marketing firm worked with a number of top-tier health care institutions, so I had some familiarity with names like Cleveland Clinic, UCLA, Mayo Clinic, University of Michigan, Johns Hopkins, and Sloan Kettering. Now, each of my Web searches yielded more granular insight on specialties, outcomes, and consumer reviews. Though I searched nationally, proximity to Saratoga Springs mattered a great deal, since it could affect whether a center was in my health plan's network. As expected, the usual suspects kept showing up in my searches, with Memorial Sloan Kettering consistently rated among the best. MSK checked a lot of boxes: highly rated cancer center, strong specialty in prostate and urologic cancers, lots of positive consumer reviews, and within a three-hour drive of Saratoga. Soon I would also learn they were in my health plan's network.

As impressive as Sloan Kettering appeared online, I admit that I harbored a bias against a New York City-based center. My professional work took me to New York frequently and my daughter attended school on the Upper West Side, so I knew the city and loved it as a place to spend a weekend, see a show, or hit the museums. But New York has an undeniable gruff side to it, and I assumed any cancer center located there would reflect that tone, to some degree. It was hard to imagine seeking care for such a sensitive health concern in a city famous for being unforgiving and impersonal. Nonetheless, the consumer reviews were encouraging, so I resolved to schedule a consultation. When I called Sloan Kettering's main number to book an appointment, I braced myself for some New Yorker attitude. To my relief, the woman on the phone was actually very pleasant. She asked about my diagnosis and any tests I had done. When I told her I was willing to consider either surgery or radiation, she offered to coordinate back-to-back appointments with a surgeon and radiation oncologist for my visit. She took down my information, asked that I send the results of my MRI when they were available, and explained how to register for the MyMSK portal, where I could coordinate appointments, research MSK caregivers, and find articles relevant to my cancer.

The whole thing was efficient and painless. Mostly, I was surprised by the difference between this phone call and my experiences with Saratoga-based specialists a month or so earlier. It never occurred to me I would be treated with more respect by a huge, New York-based cancer center than by my hometown urologist office. This was a distinction I came to see played out at every turn in my healthcare odyssey—though I kept hoping our local practitioners would eventually distinguish themselves.

The next day, I received a call from Nick, a scheduler at Sloan Kettering, who proposed some dates for my first consultation. After I chose a day that suited both Barbara and me, he gave me the names of the doctors I'd be seeing and told me where each was located on MSK's vast Upper East Side complex of buildings. He also explained that this same information would be available on the portal right after our call. And so it was, I found, complete with profiles and pictures of the two doctors, directions to their offices, and even videos to help me prepare. As a marketing communications professional, I was impressed by the sophistication of MSK's patient portal and content. And as someone who had hired scores of employees over the years, I was even more impressed by the quality of their people. Some human resources executive was on the ball down at Sloan Kettering.

Notably, both Nick and the first woman I spoke with at Sloan ended our conversations with, "Best of luck to you." It was a simple phrase, but it felt uniquely appropriate to the situation—reflecting an acknowledgment that anyone calling the center has been diagnosed with a terrifying disease. To end a call with some saccharine phrase would come across as inauthentic, but to wish someone good luck is to get the point that the patient was probably hoping for a whole lot of luck. It would be easy, even expected, for someone who spends all day on the phone fielding calls or scheduling appointments to dispense an automatic "have a nice day;" but the Sloan Kettering staff are, apparently, trained to understand that, if you just got diagnosed with cancer, you already aren't having a nice day. Maybe I'm making too much out of a single phrase, but when your emotions are raw, another person's ability to strike the right tone can be almost magical.

Scheduling with Sloan Kettering felt like a great next step for me because a single visit promised insight from two new physicians on two different courses of treatment. And at that point in my research, gaining some level of clarity was my highest priority. Having spoken to Frank and Terry, and having read about JoeBiz49's travails, I now saw prostate cancer from three entirely different vantage points, each with its unique context and nuances. While those conversations taught me a great deal, the path forward still remained stubbornly unclear. *Just give me a reliable set of facts*, I thought, *and I won't hesitate to make a decision*. As time passed, however, I was coming to believe that the set of facts I desired was a chimera. This was cancer, not a social media campaign with verifiable click-through and conversion rates. Every patient was different, every tumor its own intractable enigma. Further complicating that set of variables were the thousands of surgeons and radiation oncologists at cancer centers and small-town hospitals with skills ranging from neophyte to world-class.

Overwhelmed by all this uncertainty, I invoked Occam's razor, which instructs us that, when presented with competing hypothetical answers to a problem, one should select the answer that makes the fewest assumptions. For me, that pointed toward a place like Sloan Kettering. There, I felt, were surgeons who performed prostatectomies so often they could probably conduct the procedure on a kitchen table with a paring knife, and radiation oncologists who were literally pioneering new technologies. Additionally, centers like MSK had decades of clinical data on outcomes to give a prospective patient some statistical expectation of his own results. As icing on the cake, there was an abundance of online reviews and anecdotal feedback from patients over the course of several years. That same information was far more difficult to obtain—if it existed at all—from smaller facilities. These advantages didn't necessarily make the local urologist a poor choice; it just meant selecting one involved more assumptions than felt comfortable to me.

At least my next few steps were clear. I would travel to New York for two consultations at Sloan Kettering, and I would also meet with Dr. Z one more time to hear his treatment recommendation. Even though my confidence in him was badly damaged, he was familiar with my case, and it struck me as rash to ignore that insight. I also resolved to meet with Terry's magical surgeon in Saratoga. And, though my call with Dr. Z to discuss my MRI results had gone badly, I already knew my cancer was likely more problematic than we originally thought. This indicated that my clinical stage and Gleason score might be unfavorably revised as a consequence, and raised the ante substantially on making the right choice for treatment. With these various consultations on the calendar, I was feeling reasonably confident my treatment plan would come into focus sometime soon. One thing I knew for sure: I wanted Frank's certitude and Terry's outcome.

Most of all, though, I wanted no part of what JoeBiz49 went through.

6

THE BAD NEWS CANCER

MY FIRST APPOINTMENT at Sloan Kettering was January 17, a cold, gray Wednesday in the heart of a New York winter. Because Barbara teaches, she has the first three weeks of every January off, so we agreed to go together, meet the surgeon and radiation oncologist, and get a feel for the place. In scheduling my appointments I felt remiss for not having researched Sloan Kettering specialists myself and requested those who seemed best qualified. That would have been easier said than done— and a bit quixotic— it turns out: Sloan is a vast organization, employing over 1,000 physicians and treating more than 400 types of cancer. So I chose to believe that, based on all the information I provided, they would place me with the right people. If I didn't like their selections, I could always request someone else. Prior to my appointment, the intake professional at Sloan had requested the notes from my appointments with Dr. Z, both my PSA tests, my biopsy report, and a copy of my MRI scans when they were available. I provided all that beforehand except for the MRI, which I planned to bring with me on a CD. By the time we went to Sloan, I still had not spoken in detail with Dr. Z about my MRI results, which rankled me. I had been in touch with his office staff to request that copies of my records be sent to Sloan; and I did speak to Dr. Z briefly to let him know I was going to New York for a second opinion. He was nice enough, acknowledging the value of a second opinion, but reminded me that "we have everything you might need here to treat this." And so they did, I'm sure. It was less clear whether Dr. Z and I were a good fit. I wanted a doctor with world-class skills, patience, and empathy. And I wanted someone who treated me with respect. Maybe that was a tall order, but I had cancer, goddamnit, and I was disinclined to settle for "good enough" or "nice enough." I have never regretted taking that position.

Sloan Kettering relies heavily on its patient portal, www.mymskcc.org, to share information and coordinate patient appointments. I was told by my scheduler Nick that all my appointment information would be on the portal, including physician profiles, instructional videos, and directions to each office. Of most interest to me, of course, were the doctors I'd be meeting. So I logged in and checked them out. First, I was scheduled to meet Karim Touijer, a surgeon specializing in urologic cancers, including prostate and kidney. There was an extraordinary amount of information on Dr. Touijer, including a full profile with his credentials, a long personal statement, and even a video of him speaking about his approach. He looked about 27, though when I did the math I concluded he had to be in his forties. So I guess he had good genes. He was of Moroccan descent, apparently, having received his MD at Universite Hassan II in Casablanca. He completed his residencies at Centre Hospitalier Universitaire, the University of Kansas, and the University of Arkansas. He spoke four languages: English, French, Arabic, and Spanish. Oh, and he also had a Masters degree in Public Health from Harvard.

Definitely an overachiever. I didn't know whether to be impressed, intimidated, or contemptuous.

In his video, he spoke with a charming French accent of all the technological advancements that have made treatment of urologic cancers more effective. He had a nice manner about him—no sense of arrogance at all. I decided he looked promising.

Barbara, who also saw his video, announced that he was insanely good-looking. And so he was, I suppose. I only hoped his skills were as impressive as his accent and his ridiculously good skin.

More information on Touijer was available on the Web, including videos of him speaking (both in English and French) at conferences around the world, plus consumer reviews and papers he had authored. This was a busy fellow. I spent the most time poring over his reviews on healthgrades.com (4.7 out of 5 stars) and vitals.com (4.1 out of 5). They were impressive. Even better were the comments.

"I had my prostate removed 4/3/17. Today I went for my follow up. Cancer free. Dr. Touijer is truly a rock star. From the get go he told me exactly what was gonna happen and he nailed it."

And,

"Dr. Touijer is a lovely, kind, gentle man. He is a brilliant doctor who treated me with consideration and intelligence."

It went on and on like that. I was encouraged.

I was also scheduled to meet with a radiation oncologist named Borys Mychalczak. Aside from being scared even to try pronouncing his name, I was, frankly, terrified of anyone named Borys. I had watched too many *Creature Feature* late-night horror movies in my youth. Dr. Mychalczak, who spoke English and Ukrainian and had studied at Wayne State University, however, looked very kind and approachable in his profile photo. In his lengthy personal statement, he spoke of being in practice for thirty-three years and seeing 350 new patients a year, which impressed the hell out of me. It also saddened me to think of all those people with cancer, showing up for their radiation sessions each day with varying levels of hope. Mychalczak had a broader set of specialties, including prostate, breast, and gynecological cancers. Web searches yielded less information and fewer consumer reviews on him, though when comments were posted, they were extremely positive. Perhaps the paucity of online information on Mychalczak reflected a societal preference for the flashy surgeon over the more professorial radiation oncologists? I can't say. Maybe I was making those stereotypes up as I went. I was new to this.

From these two doctor profiles, I concluded two things about Sloan Kettering physicians. First, they are, for some strange reason, multilingual. Second, they have decades of experience and treat mind-boggling numbers of patients. I couldn't account for the first characteristic, but I liked the second. Having done my due diligence on the two doctors in question, I awaited my trip to Sloan Kettering with a mix of curiosity and anxiety. For all my exposure to cancer, my primary experiences had been limited to seeing two parents die from the disease. I had been to hospitals with oncology centers, but never to a world-class center where every patient had cancer. Nor did I know what to expect of their institutional culture and approach to patient care.

To begin with, the waiting area at Sloan's prostate cancer center is no great shakes. It's in the basement—I think they call it the "Concourse Level"—of the Sidney Kimmel Center for Prostate and Urologic Cancers on East 68th Street. My first appointment was at 9:15 AM, so Barbara and I drove to New York the night before and stayed at a nearby hotel. When we showed up for our appointment, two smiling and uniformed African-American men at the front desk directed us downstairs. I noticed, at the other end of the first floor lobby, people walking on treadmills, which struck me as odd. There were also quite a few people in the waiting area, looking like they were resigned to a long wait. The chemotherapy center, I learned later, was just around the corner, and those poor souls were waiting for loved ones undergoing treatment. As we stepped onto the elevator, it occurred to me that anyone here who wasn't a Sloan Kettering employee was most likely a cancer patient—or related to one. It was a sobering thought. When I was a child, I felt surrounded by the disease, but more on a figurative level. Now, I was literally enveloped by the physical presence of cancer—bodies standing next to me on the elevator or passing me in the hallway all carried their secret malignancies beneath sweaters and parkas, under hats and scarves. If this was a glimpse into the vast, gnostic society of cancer victims, I felt very much the novice, and it was a chastening sensation.

At the same time, I felt a growing sense of gratitude that such extraordinary institutions exist, that so many physicians' assistants, nurses, surgeons, janitors, radiologists, nurse practitioners, receptionists, anesthesiologists, and oncologists rise every morning with the sole purpose of caring for the afflicted. The previous summer, on a recommendation from

Mattie, Barbara and I had bought the audio version of *The Book of Joy*, an account of a series of dialogues between Desmond Tutu and the Dalai Lama. We listened to the book on the sixteen-hour drive back home from the University of the South near Chattanooga, Tennessee, where Barbara taught in a graduate English program. The two old, wise men have been friends for decades, apparently, and had arranged to meet for several days to discuss how one finds joy in the face of life's inevitable sorrows. It's a fascinating dialogue. The two men agree on a great deal but diverge, occasionally, on the specific methods of finding inner joy. The Dalai Lama, a Buddhist, speaks of mental discipline and keeping negative or destructive thoughts at bay through prayer and meditation. Tutu, speaking from a Christian tradition, encourages us to forgive ourselves and others, to view sadness as the foil by which we understand joy. When we listened to the book, of course, I had no idea what lay ahead. Even so, I was deeply affected by their discussion on humankind's interconnectedness, how in sorrow one can derive comfort from the presence of others who share your lot. This notion is far from *schadenfreude*, and it's not about misery loving company. It centers around embracing our shared humanity and understanding that no one suffers alone who is open to the suffering of others. We are part of a vast, connected network of humanity, the Dalai Lama intones. In that network is strength and solace.

Sitting in the crowded waiting area in the urologic cancer center, it was clear I wasn't alone. It was only 9 AM and the place was already packed, with scarcely an available seat. There had to be twenty-five or thirty people there, either patients waiting to be seen, or family members anxiously expecting the return of a father or spouse. There were men of every description, most older than I, a few younger. Most often, the men were with their wives or partners. Some were alone. Looking around at them all, I felt like we shared a common secret, that if introduced we could talk for hours about our shared experiences—all of us strangers except for the grim gift we had been given. Some of these men, I knew, were fatally ill, coming in for palliative treatment to make their remaining time more tolerable. Others, like me, were just beginning their journey toward treatment. I saw weariness, caution, skepticism, hope, anxiety, all etched on the faces in that room. And it did not undo me. In that realization, I understood, lay the first benefits of entry into the gated world of cancer.

Though the waiting area was crowded, the Sloan Kettering employees at the front desk seemed cheerful and well organized, handing off clipboards between them as patients came and went, calling out last names, showing people to their respective destinations.

"Mr. Colton?" one of the nurses called out.

An older black man rose slowly, wearily pushing himself up from his seat. He handed his parka to his wife, who accepted it with an encouraging smile. "See you in a few minutes," he muttered. I could tell he'd been there far too many times. When he approached the nurse, she didn't turn abruptly, expecting him to follow, as I'd seen countless times in the healthcare system. Instead, she watched him as he shuffled toward her, smiled, and asked, "How you doing today, Mr. Colton? You staying out of the cold?" He gave her an inaudible response and followed her in. *That nurse was giving it her best*, I thought. *Good for her.*

Before long, my name was called and a different woman greeted us just as warmly. Barbara, having just fixed herself a giant cup of tea at the refreshment station, followed me into a long hallway with what looked like dozens of examination rooms. First, we were shown into a room where they checked my pulse and blood pressure. I made some lame remark about having white-coat syndrome and the nurse laughed distractedly. Then we went to a second room where we waited for a nurse practitioner from Dr. Touijer's staff to meet with us. I was given a hospital gown that I donned with the usual resignation. I forget the name of the physician assistant, so I'll call her Rachel. I recall that she was attractive, dark-haired, friendly, and businesslike, with an athlete's gait. She began by asking me various questions about urologic symptoms and erectile function. She also asked if we had brought a copy of the MRI with us, which Barbara quickly extracted from her book bag.

"Okay, good. I'll get this loaded into the system so Dr. Touijer can get a look at it."

I asked if they could make sure Dr. Mychalczak received a copy as well; and Rachel assured me that all the doctors at Sloan Kettering had access to their centralized electronic medical records. After a few more questions about my medications list, she said she'd like to do a quick rectal exam.

What, she hadn't read the results of my 7,000 previous rectal invasions?

I assumed the squat.

I was right about Rachel's athletic inclinations. Her index finger was smaller than Dr. Quinn's, but like any athlete, she made up for size with effort, sweeping that pointer around my rear end so forcefully I think she left permanent grooves. I rocked forward on the balls of my feet, sucking in air to avoid blurting unintentional expletives.

"Well, I can't feel any nodules, so that's good," Rachel affirmed. *I could have told her that*, I thought. She snapped off her gloves and handed me a paper towel to clean up.

"Dr. Touijer should be here in just a minute. I think I heard him in the hallway." I thanked her for everything. Secretly, I wasn't sorry to see her take that nasty little finger to its next victim.

We didn't have long to wait before Dr. Touijer came in. After Rachel left, another woman stopped by to check on us and, as she was leaving, a slender young man in a royal blue suit entered the room. No white coat. No clipboard. No telltale signs this guy was a doctor. But then I saw his face and realized it was none other than the polyglot surgeon himself. It's funny—my initial reaction, and not even a conscious one, was not to like him. He was too slick, too accomplished, too good-looking. But something about his interactions with his staff suggested he was a very nice man. His team seemed relaxed around him—if perhaps a little in awe—and he showed them all respect, at one point stepping politely aside to let his PA leave the room. As he did, I took the opportunity to look him over. He was impossibly lean for a forty-something man and his meticulously tailored suit showed it— slender cut, narrow pants, coat buttoned tidily at the navel. He had dark eyes; wavy black hair; and luminous, olive skin—very much the dashing figure we saw in the video. This was a man without wrinkles or blemishes—he looked freshly made by the gods of medicine, moist with the dew of creation.

Judging from her expression, Barbara was not disappointed by Dr. Touijer in the flesh.

The doctor held out his hand and introduced himself with the same French accent we heard on the video. Then, briefly, he placed his other hand on my shoulder and said, "It's very nice to meet you, James. Let's see how we can help."

Back when I owned my marketing company, I had attended a wellness conference in Stevens Point, Wisconsin, where one of the presenters lectured about an alternative healing approach used in Hawaii. This method was ancient, he explained, and relied on human touch, especially the touch of loved ones. Wellness conferences were never my thing, I will admit, and this speaker reminded me why—way too touchy-feely for my taste. Yet, as the lecture wrapped up and he made one final demonstration, I had to concede that he struck a chord. There were roughly fifty of us in the presentation room, each sitting on a stackable conference chair and so close together that we occasionally grazed elbows. He asked us all to stand. "Now, move one step to your right and sit on your neighbor's chair."

I rolled my eyes.

For a moment I wondered laughingly what would happen when the poor lady at the far-right end of our row found herself without a seat. As I sat down, the speaker said, "Okay, now feel the warmth of your neighbor's body on the seat cushion." At first I was creeped out. But then, as he conjured visions of orchid leis and the great web of being (there was panpipe music playing as I recall), I felt oddly comforted by the presence of another human body. The speaker's point, of course, was that human touch is a potent force, and for all our intellectual and technological advances in healing, we have ignored the fundamental truth that we are animals who crave physical contact. We evolved as social beings and derive a sense of security and wellbeing from the presence—the touch—of others.

Barbara, who teaches a freshman writing course called "Tribe," talks all the time about *homo sapiens* being herd animals, of our natural desire to be surrounded by those on whom we can depend and who depend on us in return.

Fundamental to these tribal connections is close physical proximity, whether it be the campfire of the earliest humans or the shelter in which families bed down. With that proximity comes constant, incidental contact with other human beings. It reassures us that we are not alone, that we are part of a tribe or a family or a village, and should we be hurt or sick, those same physical bodies will gather around and care for us. I'm sure there is science to support the idea that physical touch reduces stress levels by releasing comforting hormones into our systems. It certainly makes perfect sense from an evolutionary perspective.

I have no idea what my stress-induced cortisol level was like when Dr. Touijer walked in, but I bet it was through the roof. And while his hand on my arm was little more than a brief reminder of our shared humanity, it also signaled that this doctor cared about more than my medical chart and made an effort, however small, to establish contact on a human level. That counted for something.

Barbara and I talked to Dr. Touijer for about thirty minutes. As you might imagine, after my diagnosis in late December we had prepared an extensive list of questions. Barbara had brought along the prostate cancer handbook Dr. Z gave me and, at one point, Touijer glanced down at the book in her hand and remarked, "Wow, you've even got the book with you! You read the whole thing?" Indeed we had. We weren't going to leave these appointments without covering everything on our list. I asked about the risks of surgery: incontinence, impotence, infections, blood clots, reactions to general anesthesia, you name it. I even broached the one subject that sent a frisson of terror through my frame: *castration-resistant prostate cancer*. The question, as I formed it in my head was, *You mean to tell me that castration is a fucking treatment for something?* However, I framed it up rather better out loud. He calmly reassured me that physical castration was rarely performed any more.

"Prostate cancer feeds on testosterone, so in more advanced cases it is helpful to eliminate the fuel testosterone provides, so the cancer can't spread as fast. Happily, there are now drugs that reduce your testosterone levels to zero while you're being treated," he explained. "They are much more effective than castration because not all your testosterone is produced in your testicles. Your adrenal glands produce a small amount as well."

As I listened, I noted to myself, *they don't cut your nuts off anymore.*

Touijer often responded to our queries by citing statistics he had compiled over years of prostatectomies. He could tell you what percentage of his patients experienced stress incontinence after six months or how many could achieve an erection good enough for intercourse. They were all very impressive statistics, derived from surveys Sloan Kettering administers before surgery and then conducts at various milestones afterward. This assiduous tracking of patient outcomes became familiar to me, as did the conditions and definitions they apply to incontinence, erections, and so forth. It is worth noting, however, that what looks like success in survey data may not align with the typical man's definition of a winning scenario. It's not that the surveys are misleading, but the clinical definition of a satisfactory erection or level of continence differs substantially from the average guy's idea of a good hard-on or a dry pair of Jockeys. But I did appreciate their strong belief in documenting outcomes.

During our conversation, Dr. Touijer also addressed my biopsy report. "I would have preferred that you had the MRI *before* the biopsy," he remarked somewhat offhandedly.

With this, Barbara looked up at him with a raptor's intensity. I knew what she was thinking.

"Really?" I said somewhat fatuously. "My urologist urged me to wait on the MRI."

"I understand he may have seen things differently," said Touijer diplomatically. "At Sloan we wouldn't have proceeded to the biopsy without an MRI. The MRI would have helped us have a more accurate biopsy—especially with your tumor, which is not as accessible from the rectum. Plus, a biopsy causes a lot of bleeding in the prostate, which can obscure your MRI images."

He went on. "It's also very unusual," he said with a mildly incredulous expression, "for a biopsy report to indicate you have an extraprostatic extension, especially when only two cores showed cancer."

Barbara and I looked darkly at each other, sensing this

wasn't a good thing. I asked Touijer to elaborate.

"Extraprostatic—or extracapsular—extension is when the cancer has pushed through the thin membrane that encloses the prostate and begins to invade the tissue outside. It's very unusual for a biopsy report to identify this," he said, "so I'm going to ask for copies of the original tissue slides so our pathologists can review those along with the MRI."

I liked that he was being so thorough, but this whole extraprostatic concept was new and troubling to me. I nervously pressed him for more details, and he was quick to assure me that, if the tumor had indeed extended outside the prostate, it was his job to remove it. "But let our people look at the MRI and biopsy slides and we'll have a much better sense."

With that, we wound down the conversation and agreed to connect by phone as soon as they had more information.

My next meeting was with radiation oncologist Dr. Borys Mychalczak. By then we had fallen behind schedule, but were assured that all appointments were updated in real time as patients moved from one meeting to another. After all, this was a place where people sometimes spent the entire day proceeding from meeting to meeting. Such is the nature of cancer: a check-in with the phlebotomist for blood work, maybe a conversation with your oncologist or surgeon. Maybe some time in chemo. Sloan was like a city dedicated to one disease, with every conceivable system to facilitate movement of patients through its honeycomb of hallways, examination rooms, and waiting areas.

Dr. Mychalczak also had a PA whose index finger I eyed warily when she came in. She was a good bit older than Rachel and, upon learning that I had already been given a "once-over" downtown, was content to consult whatever rectal health files they maintained on their computer system. She did the usual checks of blood pressure and pulse and announced that the doctor would be in shortly. Now, I will admit that I was unfairly expecting a humorless man with a thick, eastern European accent. But Dr. Mychalczak (who pronounced his name "muh-*hall*-chuck") turned out to be a cheerful man of 55 or so with white hair, active eyes, and a ready smile. Unlike his flashier colleague Touijer, Borys looked the part of a radiologist, with relaxed-fit khakis and a pair of comfortable-looking Rockports. After introducing himself, he sat down and reviewed what he knew of my cancer and what my options might be for radiation, should I decide to take that route. He noted that radiation has a different set of risks from surgery, with side effects showing up a year or more after treatment is complete. The cure rates, he confirmed, are about the same as surgery; thus, much of the decision between surgery and radiation is a matter of personal preference. Radiation is also used as a follow-up to surgery when there is concern the cancer may have spread.

"My bet," he said at one point, "is that we'll find your Gleason score is higher than a 6. That would help explain your high PSA." He paused to see if we were following his logic. "If that turns out to be the case, there's a 50 percent chance or higher you'll do radiation either as your primary course or as an adjuvant to surgery."

"You mean because a higher Gleason would suggest it's a more aggressive cancer and surgery might not be enough?" I asked.

"Yes, exactly."

I then asked him how long a course of radiation lasts. I'm thinking three, maybe four sessions under the green laser beam.

"You would come in five days a week for six weeks," he said.

I exhaled heavily.

"It's definitely a commitment of time. Many of my out-of-town patients rent apartments near here."

He was very kind, answering our many questions with great patience. Barbara and I later confessed to each other that we understood little of what Dr. Mychalczak told us: The terminology was just so abstruse, sounding more like physics than healthcare. He spoke of radioactive seeds, external beam radiation, and brachytherapy—the same language my brother-in-law Frank spoke, but even more obscure. It was all very impressive but mostly flew over our heads. Humbled, I made a note to go back and re-read the chapter on radiation therapy in our prostate cancer book. Nonetheless, I now had a decent sense of my options, with much of my decision hingeing on what we would learn from Sloan's pathology review of the MRI and tissue slides. Before I left Sloan Kettering for the day, I scheduled follow-up meetings with both Touijer and Mychalczak for the following Wednesday, January 24th.

When I got home later that evening, I made a beeline into my study and dug up the hard copy of my original biopsy report. For the entire three-hour drive back to Saratoga, it gnawed at me that I somehow missed a reference to this ominous extracapsular extension Touijer referred to in our meeting. What's more, Dr. Z had never mentioned anything about it—or not that I could recall; and I couldn't imagine ignoring such a detail if it *had* been shared. Though Touijer seemed incredulous that a biopsy could even identify such an issue, I didn't like the mere suggestion that it was possible. In my growing healthcare file, I came across a document from St. Peter's Hospital Laboratory titled "Surgical Pathology Report." My eyes moved quickly to the "Microscopic Diagnosis."

"LEFT PROSTATE BIOPSY: Prostatic adenocarcinoma, Gleason 3 + 3, histologic score 6, group 1. Tumor involves two of six cores, approximately 15 percent of the tissue present. Perineural, lymphatic vascular, and extracapsular invasion present.

RIGHT PROSTATE BIOPSY: No tumor identified."

Well, there it was—and it sounded even worse in this document than what Touijer described. Perineural, lymphatic vascular, and extracapsular invasion present. And, honestly, did they have to use the word "invasion?" It was moments like these when I could convince myself of creeping psychosomatic symptoms—faint, radiating pain in the perineum, swelling in various spots around my groin. And a very real headache exploding inside my temples. It didn't take much to get my imagination going, and this use of D-Day language about a gland the size of a chestnut only whipped me up further. Barbara hadn't been present when I reviewed my biopsy report with Dr. Z, so I couldn't say with certainty he omitted reference to an extracapsular invasion. Either way, I thought, how had this not been a bigger deal? It was a reminder, I knew, to be more proactive—to ask for copies of all my reports, scrutinize them mercilessly, ask follow-up questions, and never to drift passively in the current of the vast health care river. I needed to own the process more than I had. When I received the Sloan Kettering analysis of my MRI, I promised myself, I would be far more engaged.

As it turned out, I didn't have long to wait for that next installment in my serialized cancer adventure. Mid-morning on Friday the 19th, Dr. Touijer called. He explained that the pathology team had reviewed my biopsy slides and assigned my tumor a Gleason score of 3 + 4 = 7. It was the "good 7," but no longer a reassuring 6. Echoing Mychalczak's prediction, Touijer said this higher score correlated better to my high PSA, so they were getting a clearer picture. He assured me they would have Sloan's opinion on the MRI when I came in the following week.

My mind flashed back to the conversation with Frank and his "good 7." Frank told me that a Gleason of 7 was considered an "intermediate risk" cancer. So I wasn't in Terry's easy-breezy 6 category any more. For a moment, it occurred to me to ask Touijer if we could just believe the first pathology report instead of the new one. I liked that pathologist much better now. I also wondered if guys ever got unexpectedly good news about a malignancy. Do MRIs ever reveal that, oops, we way overestimated the size of your tumor? Or, do Gleason scores ever get downgraded to, like, a 2? With my cancer, at least, it felt like more news was bad news.

I noticed Touijer didn't sugarcoat the upgrading of my Gleason score. But he also didn't make it sound alarming. Rather, he exuded a quiet confidence that, whatever the obstacle, there was a solution. Surgeons, I've been told, often have this kind of confidence. Less generously, it's called arrogance. Either way, it seems a prerequisite for anyone crazy enough to cut open another human being's body and go poking around with a sharp knife. But Touijer's confidence didn't register with me as arrogance. He just didn't seem fazed by the challenge my cancer presented.

Later that day, Dr. Mychalczak called to pass along the same information. I explained that I'd already spoken to Touijer and expressed my gratitude that both physicians had called me just two days after my appointment to share this update. Though I could have done without the higher Gleason score, I was heartened by how Sloan Kettering conducted business.

January 24th rolled around in no time. We were scheduled to see Dr. Touijer at 11:30 AM, which meant we didn't need to drive down the night before. We got up early, bought some coffee and ham-and-gruyere baguettes at Mrs. London's downtown, and headed for New York. Having learned in the past few days that I was a Gleason 7, not a 6, and had an extracapsular extension, my hope that this would be a Terry-style cancer had evaporated. I wondered if Frank's tumor had escaped the prostate as well, and wished I had thought to ask. But as we found ourselves back in the waiting room at Sidney Kimmel, I knew I didn't have long to wait for more detail.

Moments later, we were shown to an examination room where we met Shannon, a caregiver on Dr. Touijer's team. The lingua franca of hospitals, it turns out, is your name and birthdate, which one is asked to recite every time a new person comes in or a procedure is undertaken. After confirming that I was, indeed, James Hill born April 3, 1961, Shannon asked us to sit down and proceeded to a list of questions about my health, medications, among other details. She reminded me of someone who once worked at my marketing agency, so I may have come across to her as more familiar than the circumstances dictated. *That can't hurt*, I thought. She was a slight, energetic woman with wide eyes and a capacious, toothy smile. Barbara and I warmed to her immediately. She was friendly without being unctuous, efficient without being bossy. When Shannon had the information she needed, she showed us into another room across the hall where we would meet with Dr. Touijer. Now, just to show how much I was over-analyzing things, I took an immediate dislike to this new room. Unlike the examination rooms where patients are assessed and medical mysteries explored, this room had a desk, three chairs, and a computer. It reminded me of the inevitable scenes on medical dramas when the doctor, seated behind a desk, shows the devastated patient X-rays of a chest cavity speckled with black malignancies. I didn't like the vibe at all. And I didn't trust that computer.

Before we even sat down, Dr. Touijer joined us in the room. On meeting him this second time, I noted how noiselessly he made an entrance. No slamming doors or shuffling shoes. He almost seemed to blow in with the breeze. Suited just as meticulously as he was in our first meeting, he alighted on the chair behind the desk. He explained that the Sloan Kettering pathologists had examined my MRI and he wanted to show us what they learned. Logging in to the electronic medical records system, he began sorting through various images, briefly opening one and zooming in, only to decide it wasn't the best view. Eventually he was satisfied with his choice, turned the monitor so we could see, and talked us through the results.

Holding a pen, Touijer pointed to various features he felt were significant about the tumor. Never once did he sound worried. But, consistent with our previous conversations, he never sugarcoated anything. I, of course, was on high alert to hear more about this extracapsular extension, which he addressed almost immediately. "You see this area here?" he asked with a sweep of his ballpoint pen. "This is where the cancer has pushed out of the prostatic capsule." He moved his pen again, identifying what appeared to be an entire crescent-shaped boundary along the prostate. "All along here . . . "

"That looks like a lot," Barbara said, echoing what I was thinking.

"It is," he replied. "That just means we have to cut a wider margin around the cancer to get it all." No alarm. Just that fighter-pilot confidence again.

"Does that increase the chance the cancer could spread—or has spread?" I asked.

"We always prefer to see the cancer limited to the prostate," Touijer said. "So there is some higher risk now that it has moved outside. But that doesn't mean that it has spread."

"How much higher a risk is it?" I asked, uncertain whether I wanted to hear the answer.

"I would call this a high-intermediate risk."

Talk about a show-stopper.

For a second, the room went silent. My brain, reeling from this latest revelation, sorted through the developments of the last few weeks during which I had gone from being a reassuring Gleason 6, with a small, unthreatening tumor, to a Gleason 7 that looked to have busted out of my prostate like a pitbull through a mosquito net—and I was now classified a high-intermediate risk. This whole process of learning more about my cancer was headed in the wrong direction.

Barbara didn't say anything. She sat peering at the monitor and the malevolent-looking crescent. I could almost hear her brain working as she processed this grim new information. I think my jaw was hanging slightly open in astonishment, or at least I remember it that way.

Now it was obvious to Touijer that he had us both pretty worried. Barbara resumed her furious note-taking, and the pace of her questions intensified as the news got scarier. She was kicking into wife-protector mode and it suited me just fine. What did high-intermediate mean in terms of survival rates? Did it change the likely course of treatment? Meanwhile, I had gone silent, wanting simply to crawl back into the cave of my masculine identity, throw a bear rug over myself, and pretend this whole thing was a big mistake. At one point, Touijer paused, sat back in his chair, and said, "Let me share something that might be useful for you to think about." He proceeded to explain that twentieth-century thinking about cancer viewed a malignancy as so much toothpaste in a tube: a tumor spreads because its mass takes up too much volume, which results in the cancer pushing into new areas of the body, eventually releasing cells that metastasize. As he spoke, I imagined my prostate as a tender, purple plum splitting open from unrelenting internal pressure. But more recent, more advanced theories about cancer, he continued, posited that the spread of cancer has more to do with the genetic maturity of the cancer cells than with the physical mass. The more mutated the cancer cells, the more viable they become outside the main tumor and the more likely to spread. For that reason, a Gleason 8 outside the prostate is a lot scarier than a Gleason 6 or 7. They had even seen situations where, after the main tumor was removed from the body, leaving vestigial cancer behind, the remaining tumor cells died out because they weren't genetically viable on their own.

I tried like hell to follow him as he walked through all this. He had a slight smile on his face as he talked, which I took to mean he was being encouraging. So maybe my cancer wasn't genetically developed enough to be a threat outside the prostate. I nodded hopefully.

"This is just a theory, mind you," he disclaimed.

Too late. I was already hanging all kinds of hopes on this theory of his. He had no idea of the gymnastics my mind could perform to find a comfortable narrative.

At last the conversation turned to treatment options. Eager to get some clarity on this most puzzling of questions, I asked him directly whether he felt surgery or radiation was the best option.

"Surgery can be very difficult to perform after you've undergone radiation," Touijer began. "It can be done, but it's tricky and has lots of side effects. With your situation I think surgery is the clear choice. You are young with a lot of life expectancy. You may want to have radiation as an option if the cancer returns."

"How would we know that?" Barbara asked immediately.

"PSA tests," he said. "If we get all the cancer, your PSA levels should be undetectable and stay that way. If they begin to creep up again, we'll know there are cancer cells still in there."

"And radiation would be the next step?" I asked.

"Yes, probably with hormone therapy."

Ah, hormone therapy. I remembered Frank's reference to zeroing out his testosterone. A charming prospect.

We covered more territory than I am sharing here, but the most important disclosures for me were confirmation of the extracapsular extension and Touijer's recommendation for surgery. Of course, I expected a surgeon to recommend surgery. But I was more convinced that because I might well need radiation later—a view Mychalczak shared—surgery seemed the only sensible way to go. Had I been older, radiation might have made more sense. But I was a relatively young 56. Thinking all this through, I remembered that my brother-in-law Frank was at least eight years older than I was, plus I had now leapfrogged his intermediate-risk cancer into holy shit territory, which made my case markedly different from his. Again, I was struck by how every prostate cancer is unique; and though I heard Frank's voice in the back of my head warning against the evils of dry orgasms, I could also sense the tumblers of my mental lock falling into place for surgery.

In fact, enjoying this newfound clarity about my path forward, I cancelled my follow-up appointment that afternoon with Mychalczak. From one perspective anyway, I had made up my mind and didn't want to be confused with more facts. Feeling a new sense of urgency, I set a surgery date for February 10th, and stayed in New York for the remainder of that day for a hastily-scheduled pre-surgical workup. In the course of the ensuing examination and briefing on the logistics of a radical prostatectomy, I stumbled onto a fact that astonished me: The procedure would take anywhere from four to six hours. Radical prostatectomies are, in fact, one of the most complicated surgeries to perform. That stands to reason, I suppose, given the bird's nest of highly sensitive nerves and blood vessels surrounding the prostate, *but how come that's not more widely known?* This wasn't feeling like "cancer with training wheels" anymore. What I had viewed as a largely conceptual threat now felt very near and ominous, like a mountain storm that sweeps in unexpectedly fast, pelting you with rain and hail as you run for shelter.

We didn't leave the city until 7 or so that night, by which time I had been thoroughly examined (EKG and all) and given a packet of information and bag of supplies to help me prepare. Before retrieving our car, we bought some dinner at a bodega for the long, dark drive home. Though my cancer was much scarier than before, it was a relief to have made a decision about my treatment.

I will confess that later in the week I didn't feel so certain about my choice and called Dr. Mychalczak for a brief conversation. I suppose if you let a set of facts roll around in your brain long enough, you can deconstruct any decision. He was very kind and told me he was aware I had already been scheduled for surgery. I asked him a few more questions about radiation therapy, and he patiently walked me through it all again. Clearly, he was not convinced that surgery was necessarily the superior option, but neither did he come across as disapproving. Reiterating what I read in all the literature, he reminded me that cure rates for radiation and surgery are about the same; but he also reminded me that every case is different and, ultimately, it's an intensely personal choice. I realized he was giving me permission to stick with my decision and stop doubting myself—and I appreciated his magnanimity more than I can say. With that last phone call,

I completed my fact-finding.

Having resolved to proceed with Dr. Touijer for my surgery, I made the simultaneous decision to relieve Dr. Z of any future duties associated with my care—a decision, once made, that I never looked back on with anything less than satisfaction. I likewise resolved to cancel my appointment with Terry's Saratoga Springs-based surgeon. Though he sounded like an excellent option, I couldn't imagine he was a better choice than my Moroccan *wunderkind*. I was, at last, comfortable with Touijer and Sloan Kettering and laparoscopic prostate surgery, and had no interest in disrupting that hard-won frame of mind.

What remained was to cut the fucking tumor out.

7

WAR

IT'S A HUMBLING REALITY of cancer that, for all the examinations, all the poking and prodding we do, all the X-rays, MRIs, and CT scans we endure, we never know how things *really* are inside our bodies. That's the devious thing about this horrible disease—it is the ultimate clandestine enemy. On any given evening, we watch television news stories about terrorism, reports with references to fighting a "new kind of war" or "sleeper cells" all around the world awaiting orders to activate. And that kind of war, the maddening process of tracking down an enemy that hides, strikes, and disappears again, is how they've been fighting cancer for a very long time. Terrorism scares us, particularly for its ability to materialize in places we least expect it—a nightclub in Tel Aviv, a sidewalk in Paris, a bridge in London. It is invisible and unpredictable, relying on the vastness and complexity of human existence to stay hidden until called upon to act. So much damage can be done by one man pedaling through a crowded bazaar with explosives strapped to his chest. The mere possibility of this person reminds us that any of the billions of people on Earth can unexpectedly become lethal to the rest of us, can be weaponized.

Cancer cells are the terrorists of the human body, the weaponized bundles of angry, twisted cellular matter that have come unmoored from their restraints. They, too, are created in places we cannot see, under circumstances we cannot predict. The body's immune system does what it can to detect those cells early, to catch them as they undergo their mutation, and to destroy them. It is that one malignant cell in the pancreas, brain, or breast that escapes the body's policing—for reasons science is only beginning to understand—and begins the clandestine process of forming a tumor. When a showering woman notices a lump in her breast or an elderly man feels inexplicable numbness in his fingers while writing checks, then the medical sleuthing commences to discern what form the cellular insurrection has taken. By that time, of course, the cancer cells have established a stronghold somewhere in the body from which to launch their campaign of destruction. Once the disease is identified and the treatment plan begun, it is a battle between modern medicine and its panoply of technologies and medications and the microscopic, maddeningly clever insurgents holed up deep inside the body's labyrinth of tissue, blood, and bone.

For all our twenty-first-century medical technology, there remains a medieval violence to cancer treatment—whether the body is cut open by a scalpel, irradiated by a beam, or poisoned by chemotherapy. I have to believe that, centuries from now, we will look back on our methods and wonder why some elegantly simple, non-invasive solution had not yet occurred to medicine—why hundreds of thousands of bodies were so brutalized in pursuit of a cure. Of course, the brutality of the treatments is proportionate to cancer's astonishing ability to spread, mutate, and invade healthy tissues. And with the body's own immune system—a miraculously complex and potent force—so often deactivated by cancer, how else do we eradicate such a stealthy enemy if not by extreme, aggressive measures? Perhaps immunotherapy, which awakens the hoodwinked immune system, will turn out to be that answer. Rousing the body's defenses from cancer's deception was central to my father's immunotherapy protocol published twelve years earlier, and is now proving to be a productive area of research. Until a cure is found, though, we throw everything we have at cancer treatment, accepting collateral damage to our bodies as the price of survival.

Talking about cancer in the vernacular of warfare comes naturally to anyone undergoing treatment. As much as I objected to the idea that I was "battling" the disease, I nevertheless found myself thinking about winning a war—even if that war amounted to a single skirmish played out in an operating room. Even the pathology report, as I explained previously, refers to an "invasion" by the cancer of outlying areas. It's a formidable enemy no matter how "good" the well-meaning doctor says prostate cancer is. As far as I was concerned, one cancer cell in my body was enough provocation to mount a full-on seek-and-destroy mission. And, thanks to my somehow not getting the memo that PSA tests are a good idea, I had a nastier than usual two-centimeter tumor thriving on the left side of my prostate. By the time I had received my upgraded Gleason score and been informed of the extraprostatic extension, I had developed a mounting sense of urgency. I imagine that's typical for cancer patients. After all the talk about something growing inside of you, you reach a point where you just want it out. I reached that point on January 24th, after reviewing my MRI images with Dr. Touijer.

Before prostate cancer, I had never undergone any significant surgery. My varicocele repair hardly counts, nor did the removal of a harmless lump from my left cheek. In some ways, my four colonoscopies seemed more legitimate since they involved elaborate preparation ("elaborate" applying largely to the epic consumption of lemon-flavored laxative and the subsequent and proportionate use of toilet paper) and something that felt like general anesthesia—though I'm told by the nurses I chatted up a storm the whole time. I wonder to this day what kind of dirt they have on me. All that being said, I was surprised by how much prep I was required to do for my prostate surgery. In retrospect it all makes perfect sense; that I was surprised is further proof of my naiveté about this new affliction. The thing I learned about prostatectomies, and cancer surgery in general, is they are a classic instance of "the best defense is a good offense." By that I mean the surgeon's job is to eradicate the cancer from your body. Period. Once the surgeon has opened you up, he or she goes aggressively on the offense, removing tissue where the cancer is known to be—and where it could be. With prostate cancer, the most common method for doing so is the radical prostatectomy, which involves the removal not just of the prostate, but also the seminal vesicles and nearby lymph nodes. If there is any concern the tumor has invaded the fatty tissue outside the prostate, portions of that may be removed as well. In this context, "radical" means "far-reaching" or "thorough," all this to make sure that every destruction-crazed cancer cell is removed.

After my pre-surgery workup at Sloan Kettering, I was given a white plastic bag of supplies with which to prepare for my date with destiny. Boldly printed on the bag was an MSK logo and the words, "Patient Belongings." I remember carrying that bag down Second Avenue in New York after my appointment, thinking, *well, if the world didn't know I was sick before, they certainly know now.* I might as well have worn a sandwich board. I realized that this must be the bag into which you stuff your clothes prior to surgery, a point that further drove home the reality of my situation: In two weeks, I would be unconscious for six to eight hours while my clothes sat in a plastic bag by the nurse's station, and my wife tried to keep herself distracted in a waiting area.

One of my first decisions related to surgery was that I wanted to be in excellent physical condition beforehand, so I could recover quickly. For six weeks after surgery, I was told, I was prohibited from lifting anything heavier than ten pounds, and walking would be the prescribed exercise. So I figured I'd spend a lot of time at our local YMCA getting ready for my enforced downtime. To be honest, I was also envisioning the moment when the surgical team would expose my 56-year-old abdomen for the procedure. Casual conversation among the team might ensue, I imagined, and someone would comment, "Well, here's a guy who takes care of himself." It's pathetic, I realize. But I cared. I mean, if you're going to be knocked out for hours with a cluster of people focused on your midsection, it doesn't hurt to look your best. I also wanted my abdominal muscles to heal quickly as well. So I did my Russian twists and my come-togethers, my planks and my bicycles. I toiled away on the elliptical machine watching neat drops of sweat accumulate on the control panel. I watched what I ate. I took long walks.

I also followed the elaborate instructions I was given in my Patient Belongings bag. Among other things, I was to discontinue medications, such as fish oil and aspirin, that could thin my blood; and I was to practice several times a day on my incentive spirometer. This odd device looked like a pygmy bicycle pump made of clear plastic. The purpose of the spirometer is to teach you to breathe deeply so that after surgery you can avoid having fluid accumulate in your lungs. I didn't realize it at the time, but when you have five new incisions in your abdomen, you don't tend to breathe deeply, and coughing or clearing your throat can be intensely painful. So after surgery, you use the spirometer several times a day to clear your lungs. Before surgery, practicing on the spirometer helps you form good technique and instills the habit. They call it an "incentive" spirometer because the device allows you to mark on a graduated cylinder how well you exhaled each time, so you can exceed that level on subsequent attempts. This process brought out my competitive spirit and, in the days after surgery, I would proudly show Barbara the results of my exhalations. She would smile approvingly and I would take the spirometer upstairs for another go, like a kid with a new Nintendo.

Another bit of pre-surgery preparation included practicing Kegel exercises. Now, I was familiar with Kegels after Barbara gave birth to our daughter. The exercises, I understood, would help her tighten muscles that had been stretched by childbirth. At that point my exposure was purely conceptual, but the exercises seemed like a good thing. For men, Kegels have the advantage of tightening the muscles of the pelvic floor, which control urinary function—and which are profoundly affected by a prostatectomy. The muscle you clench when you stop peeing is, essentially, the target of the Kegel exercise. The stronger you are in this regard before surgery, the better you'll regain continence afterwards. Enough said. I was all over those exercises from day one. My goal was to do three sets of ten Kegels every day, sitting, standing, lying down, whenever. The cool thing about Kegels was that I could do them without anyone knowing. One day I did three solid sets while standing in line at the post office, the only visible sign of my exertions being my finger counting, and the faraway look in my eyes. Every now and then Barbara would start a conversation not realizing I was in the middle of a set. Not wanting to lose my count, I'd politely wave her off until I finished. I think she was impressed by my dedication. It wasn't about dedication, though. JoeBiz49's experience terrified me, and I would have done anything to avoid a return trip to the surgeon or a future in diapers. By the time I went into surgery I'm certain I could have crushed a bocce ball with my pelvic floor muscles.

It is true, though, that I committed myself to being a model patient. If the nurse told me something would help my recovery, I was on it. I didn't want to be the guy who blew off instructions, only to regret it later when I blew through eight Depends a day. I wanted to get back to life as quickly and completely as possible, and if breathing into a bicycle pump or clenching my peeing muscles dozens of times a day would help, sign me up. I do think my compliance made a difference. In most respects, I had a pretty rapid recovery, hitting all the milestones they set for me.

My most intensive surgical prep occurred the night before and the morning of the surgery. We didn't know my exact surgery time but were told someone from Sloan Kettering would call by 2 PM the day before with that information. We knew it wouldn't be early morning because Dr. Touijer did only one surgery on Saturdays, which made the schedule roomier. I liked that. I wanted my surgeon well-rested, fully caffeinated, and ready to do his best work. If I was to be his only case that day, I would have his undivided attention. The Friday before my surgery, Barbara and I packed our bags and left for the City shortly after lunch. While we were in the car, I received a call instructing me to report at the hospital at 11:00 AM. *Not too late, not too early*, I thought. *Good start.*

That night, we stayed in a hotel near Sloan Kettering's Memorial Hospital where the surgery would take place. Mattie came down from Barnard and met us for dinner at a great Upper East Side restaurant. I was told to eat a light dinner, which I did, preceding it with my last cocktail for a while—a stiff Tito's on the rocks. During dinner, Mattie asked a lot of questions about how the next day would go. We explained what we knew.

I would be unconscious for seven to eight hours between prep, general anesthesia, and recovery. Barbara would be camped out in the hospital waiting room, receiving periodic updates from Touijer's nurse liaison. Sensing that Mattie was trying to figure out her role in the day, I addressed a subject that had been on my mind for a while.

"Matt," I said after a bite of hummus and flatbread, "I don't think you should come see me in the hospital."

She raised her eyebrows in surprise, as did Barbara.

"It's going to be a long day and I'll be pretty out of it after surgery. Maybe you can pop by on Sunday before we leave, or we can stop at Barnard on our way out of town."

Now, my reasoning in this instance was clear to me, but probably less so to Barbara. As a father, I didn't relish the thought of Mattie seeing me right after surgery. I would be weak, disoriented, and maybe even a little loopy. Why not have her wait until the next day when I would be more myself, more Dad-like? Perhaps that was a cop-out on my part; but having seen my mother ill for so long and my father languishing in bed before his death, I was disinclined to give Mattie hospital-bed memories just yet. In the end, both Barbara and Mattie acquiesced. Secretly, I think Mattie was relieved not to have to see me in that setting, though she never said so.

After dinner, Barbara and I sent Mattie back to Barnard in a cab, and headed to our hotel where more surgery prep awaited me. My two primary tasks that night were to shower with a powerful antiseptic soap, and to give myself an enema. As you may recall from my biopsy prep, I was now no stranger to enemas, so the concept wasn't as alarming as on my first go-round. For obvious reasons, I chose to administer the enema before the shower and was, again, successful. Feeling like a champ, I took the bottle of Hibiclens antiseptic shampoo into the shower and gave myself a long, careful scrubbing over. The pinkish liquid soap smelled medicinal and didn't generate much lather, but I could tell from the tingling on my skin that it was serious stuff. Germ-free from head to toe, I toweled off, skipped the body lotion as instructed, and headed to bed feeling scrubbed and itchy, but reasonably calm.

Around 9 AM the following morning I received another call from Sloan Kettering. Dr. Touijer was running ahead of schedule, I was told. Could I be at the hospital earlier than planned? Sure thing. I liked a doctor who was running ahead of schedule. Prohibited from eating anything that morning, I took another shower with the industrial-strength Hibiclens, dressed, packed my overnight bag, and walked over to the hospital with Barbara.

On Sloan Kettering's patient portal is posted an impressive array of instructional videos. One such video explains what will happen the day of your surgery: where to report, with whom you will meet, and how your partner or loved one will be apprised of your progress. In preparing for my surgery, I watched this video several times, scrutinizing details to anticipate how my experience would unfold. As the video begins, a young woman and her partner come strolling down the sidewalk and turn to the main entrance of MSK's hospital. She's wearing a sensible black raincoat and tall boots and carries a tidy overnight bag. Her partner is in a black jacket, jeans, and sneakers. Everybody looks comfortable and relaxed. They head to the sixth floor and check in at the concierge desk where the woman is given her wristband ID. By this point, I'm wondering what kind of cancer she has. Then I remember that she's an actor. That's not even her boyfriend. *Just as well*, I thought. *She could do better*. From the concierge desk they are shown to the Pre-Surgical Center where she is given a gown, socks, and a navy blue robe, plus a garment bag for her street clothes. She meets with various MSK staff and is then taken to the operating room. It all looks pretty well choreographed. She doesn't seem too freaked out. Her "boyfriend," looking remarkably blasé, settles down with a book in the waiting area.

All things considered, it was a pretty accurate depiction of how things go. As usual, everyone at MSK was kind and welcoming. I was shocked by how busy the place was on a Saturday. I had been expecting a more casual atmosphere with people moving around a little less urgently than on weekdays. But things were all business inside Sloan Kettering that day. You would never have known it was a weekend. Following the same steps as the woman in the video, we found ourselves in the

Pre-Surgical Center where, after the nurse closed the curtain around our space, I changed into a hospital gown, robe, and socks with rubber treads on the soles. My clothes went into a garment bag and my other items went into the now-familiar Patient Belongings bag, which we placed on the foot of the bed. A steady parade of people came and went as we prepared: a nurse or two, the anesthesiologist (very nice guy), and, eventually, Dr. Touijer. He made his usual quiet appearance, looking as serene as ever. I made a couple jokes along the lines of "Now do your best work today, okay?" He responded with the requisite laugh and headed off, I imagined, to scrub up or do whatever doctors do before a long surgery. Given that it was a four- or five-hour surgery, he was probably hitting the men's room one last time.

Seeing Touijer made the whole thing seem very real and imminent. I was pleased, though, that my nerves were not yet on edge that morning. Having gone through so much to reach this point, I believe I was content to take my hand off the tiller and drift in the current of this mighty river called Memorial Sloan Kettering. They made it easy to do so, handing you off from person to person with a combination of good manners and professional efficiency. While I was slipping into this pre-surgery passivity, Barbara, I could tell, was growing increasingly anxious. Her face was more taut than usual and her focus on every detail was intense, a sign she was uneasy. I appreciated her tiger-wife watchfulness as I readied myself for a descent into anesthesia; but it pained me to know what lay before her. At many points before my surgery and in the ensuing recovery, it occurred to me how much of cancer's burden is borne by one's partner. For all the worry, fear, pain, and discomfort the patient experiences, he has the advantage of occupying his own body, of being intimate with every physical and psychological detail in a way no one else can. One's partner can only help in limited ways yet bears the full brunt of the worry—a worry exacerbated by her dissociation from the physical experience and the resultant limits of her understanding. It's an awful place to inhabit; and as I sat there on the bed awaiting my surgery with that odd Zen-like acquiescence, regret stirred inside me like a moth's insistent fluttering against a window screen. Within minutes, my anxiety would be extinguished—temporarily, at least—by the alchemy of the anesthesiologist; but Barbara faced a solitary vigil in the lobby with only her books and magazines to distract her. As she gazed distractedly through an opening in the curtain partition, I studied the architecture of her face—the serious set of her jaw, the slender lips taut against each other—realizing, perhaps for the first time, that, though I was the patient in this story, her role was the harder one. Yet, still she presided over my illness, my body, with a fierce, unconquerable love, in return for which I could only offer gratitude.

As I sat on the bed fidgeting with the sash on my robe, Barbara listened attentively to the voices outside our enclosure. A moment later, a nurse drew back the curtain with a flourish. My chest constricted at the sound of the fabric partition sliding in its overhead tracks. Barbara looked up, fixing her gaze on our visitor. The nurse was a vivacious Hispanic woman with a big smile. She introduced herself cheerfully, asked how we were doing, and said something like, "So, are you all ready?"

Suddenly I was thinking, *hell no*. But I nodded passively, trying to recover the Zen-like state I had found earlier.

"You can either walk to the operating room or I can wheel you on the bed. Whichever you prefer," she said. I opted to be wheeled in. Somehow walking felt like a bad idea at the moment. I could imagine myself slipping on the linoleum and throwing out my knee or some other act of last-minute stupidity. I wasn't taking any chances. Plus, I felt a little shaky all of a sudden.

Distracted by my own thoughts, I turned to Barbara for a goodbye kiss and saw that her eyes were pink and welling with tears; big, wobbly drops clung tentatively to her lower eyelashes. Moved by her sudden vulnerability, I reached for her hand. It was all I could do at that point. My ability to console anyone was, at least for the moment, suspended. I was a patient about to be wheeled off to surgery. She, in turn, faced the equivalent of a workday alone in the hospital lobby. There was nothing to say, and we both knew it.

"Don't worry," the nurse exclaimed. "He's going to be fine."

"I know . . . " Barbara looked down, her voice trailing off uncharacteristically. I squeezed her hand. Now I was getting a lump in my throat.

"He's got a great surgeon," the nurse continued. "Dr. Touijer is amazing."

"Is he?" Barbara smiled hopefully. We were both keen to hear anything encouraging about the man who would be rooting around in my reproductive and urinary systems.

"Oh, he's incredible. Everyone here loves him." Then, spontaneously, the nurse came over and gave Barbara a hug. It wasn't a big, flashy moment by any means—just a woman whose humanity was alive and well that Saturday morning; and in the midst of her getting a patient to his prostatectomy, she let the anguish of another human being make her pause.

Then Barbara drew back her shoulders and took a breath as if to say, "Okay, you can have my husband now." She stepped back to let the nurse steer my bed out of our cubicle. I don't remember exactly how we lost eye contact or what her expression was the moment I was wheeled away. I only remember how intensely I felt her presence—her powerful vigilance—radiating from her like heat from an idling car. Grasping that sensation for the brief moment it lasted, I turned my gaze down the hall.

Several automatic double doors later, I was wheeled into Main Operating Room 9. I knew intellectually that a prostatectomy was a big deal; but seeing the array of people and technology gathered in that room, focused entirely on the malignant gland in my groin, I was impressed with the gravity of the moment. There had to be six or more people milling about, preparing machines, looking at monitors, adjusting instruments. The room was big, brightly lit, and surprisingly cold. I was asked to move off my rolling bed onto a heated bed for surgery, after which two nurses fastened a safety strap around me and arranged my blanket to make me warm. It was all a bit overwhelming, but the OR nurses were so efficient I scarcely had time to get anxious. Just as my body registered the warmth of my heated bed, someone clipped a monitor on my index finger. Seconds later, the anesthesiologist, whom I had met in the Pre-Surgical Center, came over and said something about going to sleep.

It was ironic, I thought later, that this war I chose to wage began not with a defiant cry or rush of goosebumps along my limbs.

Instead, it commenced quietly, with the oblivion of anesthesia, the black, utterly dreamless negation of consciousness that modern pharmaceuticals induce. It is astonishing that a human body can be so physically manipulated, shaved, cut, prodded, and stitched over the course of hours, while the brain slumbers so deeply not a single touch of the scalpel or prod from the laparoscopic trocar can disturb it. In the days before my surgery, I read terrifying accounts of people who, because of some error in the cocktail of drugs prepared by the anesthesiologist, become fully conscious halfway through their surgery. One BBC article titled "Waking Up Under the Surgeon's Knife" had a particularly gripping effect on me: A woman undergoing exploratory laparoscopic abdominal surgery woke up just before the surgeon made his first cut. Because she had been given a paralytic drug, she could not speak or move her body to indicate she was conscious; but she was completely alert and able to feel everything that occurred during her ninety-minute procedure. How could anyone survive such agony? Traumatized by this possibility, my macabre imagination turned to the revenge flick Law Abiding Citizen. Gerard Butler's character, whose wife and child are brutally murdered in his presence, exacts a creative but chilling revenge on their killer. He tracks the man down, injects him with a paralytic drug to immobilize him—and a stimulant to keep him awake. Then the "law-abiding citizen" straps his wide-eyed but helpless victim to an "operating table" where he employs pliers and circular saws to take his long-awaited revenge. These were the paranoid musings of a prostate cancer patient with anxiety and a bad case of insomnia. Happily, my terrified ruminations on paralytic drugs and anesthetic awareness passed quickly. In Operating Room 9, I felt remarkably safe and calm when the anesthesiologist strapped the oxygen mask over my mouth and nose. During my varicocele surgery many years before, the anesthesiologist had told me to count backwards from 100. The Sloan Kettering anesthesiologist made no such request. I wouldn't have made it to ninety-eight.

Whatever they dripped into my IV that day was so instant, so complete, that my brain didn't so much as sputter until about 6 that evening. I blinked into consciousness like an old computer starting up, haltingly, laboriously searching its systems to make sure everything was more or less functional. Eyes open and straining to focus, I found myself in a curtained area like the Pre-Surgical Center where I began my odyssey that morning. I was alone but could hear voices nearby as caregivers went about their business. My first real physical sensation was a sharp pain in my left shoulder. This wasn't entirely new to me: I had tears in both my left and right labrum and consequently felt discomfort when I overdid military presses or throwing the football. Why my shoulder should hurt after prostate surgery, however, escaped me. But I wasn't thinking clearly about anything yet. My mind was still stumbling into consciousness.

Nurses were talking to each other outside my curtain.

Cabinets opened and closed.

I began to feel stiffness in my abdomen, but because I was lying still, it wasn't uncomfortable so much as, well, there.

Someone swept open the curtains to my enclosure. It was a youngish man in a white medical coat. He introduced himself as a "fellow" in urology and asked me how I was feeling.

"My shoulder hurts like hell," I said. My mouth and throat were dry and words came out with difficulty.

He laughed and said something like, "Well, if that's our biggest problem, you're doing well."

I still wanted to know why my shoulder hurt.

At some point a few minutes later I heard a nurse saying something about my being awake. Then I heard Barbara's voice. The curtains opened again and a nurse in blue scrubs walked in followed by Barbara. I don't remember our reunion too well. Barbara described me as being loopy, the way I was after my colonoscopy. "You were sweet, though," she told me, "and very talkative." She noticed that my face was swollen, particularly my lips and around my eyes, but otherwise, she said, I looked reasonably good. I remember sensing Barbara's relief and wondered how tough it must have been for her to wait around all day. She asked how I felt and whether I was in any pain. Aside from my damn shoulder, I said, I felt pretty good. Hearing this, the nurse explained that my position during surgery may have extended my arm in a way that strained the tear in my labrum. She also told me that, during laparoscopic surgery, they fill your abdomen with air which, strangely, can result in shoulder pain as it moves around inside your body. I hadn't heard about the inflation concept and imagined with disappointment my bloated abdomen under the surgical lights like a beached dolphin. *So much for all that ab work,* I thought.

Turning from my sore shoulder to the surgery itself, I asked Barbara what news she received from Touijer. I was too tired and woozy to be anxious. I just wanted to know. "He said everything went exactly as expected," she replied with visible relief. "There were no surprises at all." The next day when I was more lucid, Barbara explained how her day had passed while I was in Operating Room 9. After giving her cell number to the nurse liaison for periodic updates on my surgery, she settled in to a waiting area to catch up on reading for her courses. Her distractedness was so complete, however, that she mostly sat there in a haze of worry and absent-mindedness. Every sixty to ninety minutes she'd get a call from the nurse liaison who told her how surgery was proceeding. When there was new information to share, Barbara would dutifully thumb-type text updates to Mattie and all eight of our combined siblings, many of whom were checking in during the procedure. At some point, she tried the food in the cafeteria and concluded that, for all Sloan Kettering's virtues, the hospital's cuisine wasn't at the same level as its healthcare. At about 5 PM, six hours after we had parted in the Pre-Surgical Center, she was notified that the surgery was over and Dr. Touijer was available to debrief her. Suddenly roused from hours of desultory half-reading, Barbara piled her things into her book bag to go.

At the reception desk upstairs, she was greeted by a nurse and shown into a hallway where she encountered Touijer, still wearing his surgical scrubs, sitting on a countertop and looking at his smartphone, his legs dangling casually like a restless kid in a church pew. Barbara remarked to me later that he looked as fresh as when he'd greeted us in the morning—no sweat streaks down the back of his scrubs, no stubble on his face, no eyes bleary from peering for hours into a computer monitor. Far from exhausted, he looked like he had slipped into the hallway for a quick game of Candy Crush. Barbara decided that a five-hour surgery must be just another day at the office for Touijer—and if my surgery was so effortless he didn't break a sweat, it had to bode well for the outcome. In fact, we learned later, Touijer performed four to six prostatectomies every week—and 150 to 200 per year. It *was* just another day at the office.

As Barbara approached, Touijer looked up from his phone, smiled, and greeted her warmly. With a reassuring hand on her back, he showed her into a nearby office where he carefully explained the details of my surgery. This was the part where I probed her on specifics. Chagrined, she admitted she was so relieved to hear things went well that she didn't ask many follow-up questions.

I understood that completely. I would have reacted the same way.

"He told me we'll know a lot more when your pathology report comes back in a couple weeks," she explained.

"He wasn't surprised by anything he saw in there?" I asked.

"No. He said it went exactly as he expected."

That was good enough, then. As long as Touijer was encouraged and Barbara was relieved, I was satisfied.

The night after my surgery was a blurry, jumbled affair. The remaining effects of the anesthesia were powerful and I was overwhelmed by a pervasive drowsiness. Most of the time I was content to lie in my bed and drift in and out of sleep. After some initial uncertainty whether I would be given a private room or spend the night in my curtained cubicle, we were told I was being moved to the nineteenth floor. Judging from the nurse's description, this was a bit of good luck. Eventually I was moved upstairs into a nice, quiet room with a television, an upholstered chair, and a view toward the East River. Various nurses came to check on me, noting my oxygen levels, taking urine samples from a catheter bag hanging on the side of my bed, and emptying a clear plastic bulb hanging from an incision in my abdomen. At one point, I peeked at my midsection and groin, bracing myself for what I expected would look like a war zone. It wasn't so bad. There were five or six gauze bandages taped over incisions—but nothing huge and no sign of blood. Farther down my groin, I could see the Foley catheter extending from my insulted-looking penis. The tube ran down my left leg to a plastic clip on my thigh, which had been shaved smooth, then disappeared in the darkness of my covers. Clearly this was a body after surgery, but it wasn't as shocking as I expected. There was more skin than bandage.

At around 7 or 8 PM, seeing that I was exhausted and ready to sleep, Barbara bade her farewell and headed back to the hotel. She conferred with the nurse on when to return in the morning and, with a fragrant kiss to my forehead, gathered her things and left. Throughout the night, various people appeared in my room, logging into a computer on a moveable cart. They would record my vital signs, check my catheter bag, empty something that looked like red Jell-O from the plastic bulb hanging from my abdomen (I learned it was called a Jackson Pratt Drainage System and removes bodily fluids from the surgical sites), and generally check me out. The room was dark enough for my addled mind to sleep, though never deeply. The computer monitor glowed all night, as did some kind of night light on the wall behind my head. Under normal circumstances, all these distractions would have driven me nuts: I'm a light sleeper with particular sensitivity to light. But I was still pretty doped up from the residual effects of the anesthesia, and slumber came easily.

One of the people who tended to me during the night was an older black man whose name I can't remember, so I'll call him Lawrence. He wore spotless white from head to toe and spoke kindly but a little dictatorially, with a melodious Haitian accent. I gathered from the way he went about his work that he was a longtime Sloan Kettering employee who brought military-style discipline to his caregiving—and expected the same from his co-workers. He talked as he worked, though I couldn't tell whether he was addressing me. In the darkness of the room, he would move about my bed, his white clothing glowing softly in the light of the nearby computer.

"Good, good," he'd say, to no one in particular.

Then, looking at how my catheter tube was clipped to the bedside, "No, this is not right at all."

I liked his manner immediately, and when he me asked me to sit up or roll on my side, I followed his instructions with the obedience of a first-grader. On his second visit to my room, Lawrence turned up the lights and whispered, "It's time for you to get up and do some walking around." It felt like the middle of the night and I was consequently disinclined to go do anything other than sleep. He corrected me that it was still relatively early, though my anesthesia told me otherwise. "I'll help you get up and get going," he said as he removed my covers. Seeing I had no choice, I figured I'd get it over with quickly, so I could get back to sleep.

As Lawrence helped me get positioned to sit up and swing my legs off the side of the bed, I realized why this was a big milestone. Sitting up requires abdominal strength; and I had five new incisions that made the slightest engagement of my core muscles an agonizing affair. Instantly realizing that I needed a lot of help, I submitted to Lawrence's ministrations, listening to his every instruction on where to put my elbow or how to move my hips. With his help, I sat up and, with even more assistance, swung my legs to the side of the bed. Gripping anything that came in handy, including Lawrence at various points, I eased my feet to the floor, straightened my legs, and paused, already exhausted. Holy shit. I felt like a fawn wobbling on unsteady legs.

"You're still feeling the anesthesia," Lawrence reminded me. "It's very, very powerful, but it will be worn off tomorrow." He positioned the stand holding my IV and catheter bag, explained how to grip it as I walked, and encouraged me to get going. I took a few tentative steps and realized that my biggest risk was being so unsteady. I imagined getting dizzy and toppling over in the hallway, the IV stand crashing down as I went. I knew I looked pathetic at that point—hair rumpled up, stubble of beard, hospital gown loosely tied in the back—but I was too tired to give a shit. I went through the door and into the hallway. With each laborious step, I felt a little steadier on my feet. This was when I realized how luxurious the nineteenth floor was. The halls were wide, carpeted, and nicely lighted. Expensive-looking artwork lined the walls. As I passed other rooms, I peeked in to see what looked like hotel rooms with incandescent lamps, upholstered furniture, and flat screen televisions. I remarked to Lawrence how posh the place was.

"You are very lucky to be on this floor," he whispered. "This is where they put celebrities when they come for treatment. The Shah of Iran was treated here."

"Really?"

"Yes, he had a huge security detail that stayed with him the entire time," he continued. "They also have actors and athletes who come here in complete secrecy."

Hearing all this, I was feeling fortunate for my room assignment, though I had no idea how I ended up on the celebrity floor. Maybe Barbara had employed her fierce negotiation skills to secure this room while I flickered in and out of consciousness. I proceeded to the end of the hall, at which point I felt a powerful wave of nausea suddenly rising inside me. When I signaled my distress to Lawrence, he helped me back to my room. Once I was seated on the side of my bed I told Lawrence I had to vomit. Now. He grabbed a plastic tub from the bathroom and held it under my chin.

"The nausea is from the anesthesia. Go ahead and vomit," he said. "You'll feel much better."

There was no lack of enthusiasm for letting loose at that point, but each time I retched, my abdomen exploded in pain. Up inside me the nausea welled, and over and over again I retched, only to be held back by spear jabs to my torso. It was a horrible predicament, my body wanting desperately to be rid of whatever toxic residue was pooling in my stomach, my mind unwilling to let go for fear of the agony that awaited every twinge.

So this is hell, I remember thinking.

After several minutes of violent dry heaves, the nausea subsided. Disappointed I hadn't been able to vomit, Lawrence helped me back into bed, rearranged my covers, and positioned my catheter bag. By the time he dimmed the lights and left, I was drifting off again.

Some time during the night, Lawrence was replaced by a slightly gruff woman whose name I have forgotten. She was capable but unfriendly. At around 1 AM she woke me and asked if I had seen the educational video on catheter care (a skill I would need in the coming week). Irritated by her timing, I replied that I had not. "Do you want to watch it now?" she asked, apparently unaware that, for some people, it wasn't the middle of the work day.

"I'll watch in the morning."

Reluctantly, she backed off and I went back to sleep.

And so the night proceeded, with checks taking place seemingly every few minutes. In the morning, my mind was considerably clearer, though my aches and pains were more pronounced. I devoured my breakfast, not having consumed anything in the last 24 hours other than sherbet and apple juice before bedtime. Then I lingered over my coffee while the nurse readied the infamous catheter care video for me. Barbara arrived around 9 and sat with me while we waited for me to be discharged. I was instructed to take another walk, which I accomplished with considerably more energy than the night before. The hallway of the nineteenth floor is a long rectangle around which prostatectomy patients are instructed to take as many laps as possible. At any hour of the day, you will see men and women wearing either hospital-issue gowns or, for those better prepared than I, their own pajamas or bathrobes. They push their IV stands along with them. Some shuffle along in obvious pain. Others make a show of feeling hardy by moving purposefully past room after room. On my circuit that morning, I observed a woman who, I could tell, was no stranger to Sloan Kettering. She was wearing her own bathrobe and moved through the hallway as if she owned the place. But she was also clearly in pain, never smiling or saying hello, focusing solely on putting one foot in front of the other. Every now and then I saw her husband walking with her. They moved together in silence, their faces haggard—*the faces of cancer,* I thought, *each suffering in his or her private way.*

On my second or third lap around the floor, I saw a man, dressed in a pale-blue gown just like mine, wheeling his IV stand down the hall in my direction. As we approached each other, he caught my eye. "Morning!" he called out. I slowed my approach and returned the greeting. He was an odd-looking but amiable fellow. I guessed he was in his mid-sixties, but he had a youthful charisma about him. He had a remarkable head of wavy gray-brown hair with tight curls obscuring his hairline . . . like of wisteria hanging over a balustrade. His most notable features, though, were his gibbous, strikingly blue eyes that darted back and forth between Barbara and me as he spoke. He had a carefully clipped moustache, as well, which, coupled with his coiffure, made me wonder if he was a stage performer of some kind. "In for prostate surgery?" he asked, catching sight of my catheter bag. I affirmed that I was.

"Me too! Who was your surgeon?"

"Karim Touijer."

"Ah," he nodded with approval. He told me the name of his surgeon, which didn't ring a bell. Over the next few minutes we chatted about Gleason scores, PSA numbers, and our respective experiences with surgery. I couldn't help but like him. He had a bouncy energy and punctuated our conversation with encouragement like "You're looking great!" and "Jeez, you're walking like you never had surgery!" I found myself encouraging him in return, as if reaching the tacit understanding that buoying your fellow cancer patient is essential. We talked a few more minutes and resumed our circuits, heading in opposite directions. I passed him a couple more times, and each time he politely asked another question, which would ignite another brief but friendly exchange. The last time I passed him, I wished him well, adding, "Hey, maybe we'll run into each other when we come back for our six-week PSA tests."

"That'd be great!" he beamed. "Hey, God bless. Be well."

"You, too."

I never got his name. But he was just the right person to connect with that first morning after surgery. I don't know where he found his energy or his optimism, but it was contagious; and I was glad to have met him.

In fact, six weeks later, I was having lunch in the Le Pain Quotidien restaurant near Sloan Kettering when I glanced across the restaurant at a couple just sitting down to eat. Sure enough, there he was, with his unmistakable blue eyes and curly hair. Barbara and I were just finishing, and as we rose to leave, I crossed the restaurant to where he and his wife were sitting. "Hi. You may not remember me, but . . . "

"Saratoga Springs!" he exclaimed, his eyes glinting like marbles.

"Wow! Yes! How are you? In for your PSA?"

He confirmed that he had given blood that morning and was staying in town to consult with his surgeon on the results. Barbara and I lingered by their table for five minutes or so and we shared war stories about our recovery. Things had gone well for him and he was confident his PSA test would be good news. "I'm sure it will be," I affirmed in my best, most optimistic tone. As we got ready to part ways, I expressed how pleased I was that we crossed paths again. He was still sitting as Barbara and I buttoned up our coats to go. He leaned over, put a hand on my forearm and squeezed it. "God bless you two." Then, as if the thought sprang into his mind urgently but unexpectedly, he said in a surprisingly serious voice, "We're lucky guys, aren't we?"

"We are," I said. "We really are."

As I walked away, I found myself ardently hoping he would receive good news that day—that he would be as lucky as he felt. Somehow he just deserved that.

They kept us at the hospital until lunch time. We were briefed on my pain prescriptions, how to manage the Foley catheter (my new companion), when to remove the gauze pads on my incisions, and other medical details. Mid-morning, a nurse came by to check the Jackson Pratt drainage bulb hanging on my left side. It had only a little of the bright red fluid in it; and when the nurse looked it over, she expressed satisfaction with my draining.

"Do I keep this thing on when I go home?" I asked cautiously.

"No, we can take it out right now, in fact."

With that she reached down, made a couple preparatory adjustments to the bulb and said, "This is going to feel a little strange, but it comes out fast." Now I had no idea exactly *what* comes out, so there was no way to anticipate the sensation. I quickly realized the bulb had an extremely long tail—a flexible tube about a foot long, attached to a drainage end that sucks up fluid from the surgical site. With a single pull of her hand, this entire apparatus snaked its way across the inside of my abdomen and out the inch-long incision. It happened fast, but it was uncomfortable and unnerving to feel a foreign object exiting my body, like an earthworm abandoning its tunnel. As quickly as she extracted the tube, she threw it in a waste receptacle and taped some gauze to the incision. It occurred to me that, unlike a pregnant mother who feels a baby kicking beneath her skin, I've never felt something moving *inside* my body. Yet another first in my strange cancer journey.

Next, the nurse removed the IV port on my hand, applied a gauze, and wrapped my hands with stretchy medical tape so that I looked like a boxer with his gloves off. After she left, Barbara helped me gather my things and pack up my bag. In went my medications and instruction print-outs. In went my catheter supplies, including my "night bag," dozens of sterile moist wipes, little packets of lubricating jelly, and other such accoutrements. Then I got dressed into my street clothes, which took some maneuvering since I now had a catheter bag strapped around my left calf. Having been advised to bring loose-fitting pants, I slipped into a pair of favorite black joggers, which did a good job of hiding the catheter tube slanting from my central plumbing down across my thigh to the top of the bag. When I was finally dressed I looked more or less normal—banged up as hell and in need of a shave, but functional.

Barbara snapped a picture of me to send to our two families. Looking at the image these months later, I now see how tired I was. In the picture I'm holding up my "boxer" hands, smiling bravely for my siblings to let them know I was on the road to recovery. Picture taken, we grabbed our bags and headed for the lobby. Barbara carried anything that was slightly heavy since I was prohibited from lifting much of anything. While Barbara went downstairs to retrieve the car, I milled around the nineteenth-floor reception area, admiring the artwork that lined the hallways, most of which appeared to have been donated by wealthy Sloan Kettering patients. Now I understood how grateful patients must feel after the emotionally intense experience of surgery. Though my stay had been brief—almost exactly twenty-four hours—I had never in my life been the subject of such intensive focus, so much concerted caregiving. And though I knew I was just one of hundreds of patients who would course through the hospital that month, I still felt a powerful sense of intimacy and gratitude for the staff who cared for me. I was inclined to send a thank you for the care I received, but it would be a basket of fruit or a handwritten card rather than a collection of Mapplethorpe prints, as one donor had provided. I wandered around slowly for fifteen minutes or so, getting used to wearing a catheter, feeling happy to be up and out of bed. A woman at the reception counter asked if she could help with anything.

"No thanks," I said. "I'm just waiting for my ride."

"Going home today?" she said, "Well, best of luck to you."

A moment later, Barbara called to let me know she was waiting out in front of the hospital. A nice, heavyset nurse accompanied me to the elevator and down to the front entrance where Barbara was waiting by the car. It was a cold, gray February day and Barbara's breath plumed before her as she waited. She helped me situate myself in the car without exerting my shell-shocked abdominal muscles. Inside the car I gave a sigh of relief to be done with surgery—but just as much from a sense of physical depletion.

Barbara and Mattie had conferred that morning and decided it didn't make sense for us to stop by Barnard on the way out of town. They agreed instead that we'd see each other later in February or early March. With that decision made, we had only to make the three-hour drive back to Saratoga Springs, which Barbara undertook with supreme care, avoiding potholes and bumps in the road to spare my tender midsection and groin. Just after dark, we pulled up in front of our gray and white Dutch Colonial. As usual, there was a two-foot berm of dirty snow along the road, and ice on the sidewalk, so Barbara helped me pick my way from the car to the front door. Once inside, we ate a light dinner and watched the evening news. By 9 PM I was more than ready to turn in.

I remember trudging up the stairs like an 80-year-old man with bad knees. Our house dates to 1907 and every part of it creaks, most of all the stairs. As I ascended, each step gave its own plaintive groan, articulating the self-pity I'd been fighting all day. After brushing my teeth I sat down to change my catheter from the strap-on day bag to the more capacious night bag. Never having done this before, I was all thumbs, trying desperately to recall the video they showed me at the hospital. Worst of all, I was utterly humiliated. I thought of when Barbara's father, dying from Parkinson's disease, had been catheterized and the amber bag of urine had hung from the side of his hospital bed. Now, here I sat on the edge of the bathtub, fumbling around with this new bodily attachment, feeling decrepit and embarrassed. When I grumbled about my reduced state, Barbara reassured me, "I don't see you as pathetic at all. You've been a warrior today."

Eventually, I figured out the catheter situation and made my way to the bedroom, the night bag clutched in my right hand like a briefcase, its tube disappearing into my underwear. Slowly, cautiously, I sat down on the side of the bed. Barbara hung the catheter bag on the bed frame and clipped the tube to the contour sheet to ensure that gravity did its job in directing urine away from me into the bag. But when it came time to swing my legs into bed, I realized with dejection that I couldn't do it. I was as feeble as an infant, depleted from surgery and medications, and tired out from our three-hour drive. Every effort to recline my upper body or to bring my legs up on the bed was met with stabbing pain in my midsection. After several frustrating attempts, despair welled up in me like a pool of black water. "Fuck," I muttered to myself.

Barbara stood by patiently, letting me collect myself for another try.

"I can't believe how weak I am."

"You'll get it," she replied.

As I sat there, trying to figure out how to simply lie down, I got a glimpse into the darkest chamber of cancer's secrets. I knew I was trespassing in a way, and had no real claim to this knowledge. After all, I hadn't been through countless surgeries, undergone months of chemotherapy, or submitted to weeks of radiation. I was a mere novitiate with no claim to great suffering. Yet, in that moment of weakness and fear, I felt the shadow of cancer's hopelessness pass over me like a bat flitting across an evening sky. How many patients, I wondered, reached a point where life was merely a succession of days filled from morning to night with worry, pain, exhaustion? For them, I could imagine, death seems not a plunge into a terrifying chasm but a release, an unburdening from the agonizing labors of living. Strangely, for all my frustration and self-pity with having been so depleted by this diagnosis, I was grateful for that glimpse at cancer's endgame. Both my parents, I am certain, reached the point where life just didn't seem so precious anymore and not even their children gathered at the bedside could restrain them from taking the gentle fall backward into night. For the first time, I experienced on a visceral, existential level the reality of cancer. The thought chastened me.

I sat there on the side of the bed, aching in every part of my body, terrified by my own fragility.

"I'm too weak, Barb," I said. "You're going to have to help me." And so she did, lifting my legs onto the bed and easing me back down onto the pillows. As I settled in, the shadow passed and my spirits revived somewhat. The surgery had gone well, I reminded myself. Until someone told me otherwise, I could expect to get better, for tomorrow to be brighter than today. With the presence of the catheter, I could only lie flat on my back, which wasn't my customary sleeping position. Normally that would have kept me from sleeping. But that evening, all bets were off. I didn't fall asleep so much as let myself recede, my consciousness slowly atomizing in the quiet darkness.

"Good night, warrior man," Barbara said from above me in the shadows.

Feeling more vanquished than victorious, I thanked her for all she had done. I'm not certain I finished my sentence.

8

FREEDOM

FIFTH AVENUE IN SARATOGA SPRINGS is a broad tree-lined street that, at its eastern terminus, t-bones abruptly into Henning Avenue. On the north side of Fifth Avenue, just before the Henning intersection, is a Methodist Church, a tidily maintained but sprawling modern structure of brown brick. Surrounding the church are expansive parking lots where Mattie and I rode our bicycles when she was a little girl. It was a good out-and-back course for therapeutic walking: From our house to the church it was a straight shot down the lightly traveled stretch of Fifth Avenue, and then a return by the same route, the whole excursion totaling about two miles. It was a mid-February day when I was out walking this route and, as usual, Saratoga greeted me with a slate-gray sky and temperatures in the 20s. I was dressed for warmth, comfort, and anonymity: loose joggers to hide my catheter bag, my favorite Asics tennis shoes, a blue parka, and wool gloves. To avoid being recognized by neighbors or engaged in conversation by passers-by, I wore wrap-around sunglasses and a wool baseball cap. With my short beard, I figured, I was pretty much unidentifiable.

Just before the entrance to the church, there is a wide shoulder on the left side of the road where, in the summer, grass mingled with crumbling asphalt. On this winter day, it was an expanse of brittle ice and gravel. It was an auspicious location for my purposes. Looking around to make sure there were no cars or pedestrians approaching, I paused there and, pretending to pull up my left sock, lifted the hem of my pants a few inches, identified the end of my catheter bag, and snapped it open. I waited a few seconds to let the bag empty and closed it just as cleverly. Except for some rising steam and a hole melted in the ice near my foot, no one would know I had just relieved myself outside a church.

The days immediately following my surgery became a pretty predictable affair. I would rise in the morning and head into the shower with my night bag. There I would position my face toward the shower head and let the hot water course over my face, down my chest, and over the five incisions on my abdomen, each wound secured by a two-inch-long Steri Strip. Showers had a near-miraculous effect on me, rinsing away what felt like a night-long accumulation of post-surgical detritus, and soothing the stiff muscles around my midsection. After shaving, I'd change to my day bag, dress in one of several pairs of loose-fitting athletic pants, and head downstairs for a day of reading, taking walks, and emptying the Camelbak on my left calf. Knowing I would have the catheter removed in about a week made the whole thing tolerable. Just as important, I discovered little tricks I could employ to make myself more comfortable, enabling more activity and longer walks. Within a few days after surgery I was logging over 10,000 steps on my FitBit exercise tracker and feeling a steady return of my stamina. Every now and then I'd take a selfie while out on a walk and send it to Mattie with a caption like "Crushing it today!!" followed by an emoji of a flexed bicep. It had been a long slog since my night at Sloan's Memorial Hospital—or even since my first outing at home, when I walked half a block before turning back from exhaustion. I was proud of my progress and looked forward to having the catheter removed and getting back to a more regular lifestyle.

Before surgery, I think I dreaded the catheter more than any other aspect of recovery. And it was, indeed, an uncomfortable inconvenience. When I bent over to tie my shoe, the tube running up my urethra into my bladder bent awkwardly, creating an unpleasant pressure deep in my lower abdomen. Depending on how the tube was positioned in my underwear or whether I had applied sufficient lubrication where the catheter extended from my manhood, I sometimes cut a walk short to make tactical adjustments. And, because the day bag was designed for mobility and not volume, I found myself emptying it constantly. I was prohibited from driving while the catheter was in, which didn't matter much since I was disinclined to venture out in public anyway. Mostly I stayed around the house, reading, watching television, and taking walk after walk after walk.

The long-awaited catheter removal was scheduled for February 19th, nine days after my surgery. That event was to coincide with receiving my surgical pathology report, which, of course, terrified me. The report, which assessed actual tissue samples from my surgery, would reveal how well Dr. Touijer had succeeded in rooting out the insurgency in my prostate, and whether there was a likelihood that any cancer remained. My previous consultation with Touijer, along with my subsequent reading, underscored the ominous significance of phrases like "positive surgical margins" or "involvement" of lymph nodes or seminal vesicles. Talking to us before my surgery, Touijer had clarified that "This is one place where 'positive' is a bad thing. We want to see *clear* surgical margins." Knowing that I had an extraprostatic extension, a Gleason of 7, and a high-intermediate risk, I was at least intellectually prepared for the possibility I might need a second round of treatment, most likely radiation. Being a realist, I had rehearsed this likelihood to myself for two weeks, though in my deepest inner sanctum of hope, there was no acceptance of it.

Tens of thousands of FitBit steps later—and countless trips to the bathroom to empty my day bag—I was back at Sloan Kettering waiting to see Shannon, Touijer's always-upbeat nurse practitioner. Barbara was with me and, though I knew she shared my anxiety about the pathology results, her face registered more determination than fear. She had an impressive ability to fix in her mind a positive outcome, effectively eliminating all other unsatisfactory potentialities. I had no such ability and had, consequently, availed myself of a Klonopin that morning. Even with the help of the yellow pill, my heart was thudding away and my breathing was stubbornly shallow. Having Barbara there helped calm me, though. Since receiving my initial diagnosis without her in the room, I had learned the value of her presence when I received important news. Other cancer survivors have since reinforced that sentiment to me: It's nearly impossible, they all agreed, to listen well when your autonomic nervous system is in all-out rebellion. Have someone present to do the listening for you, to ask questions and take notes while you stare blankly at the tile floor trying to clear your head. Plan for the inevitable anarchy in your anxious brain.

Such was my state of mind when the door swung open and Shannon walked in, all smiles and efficiency. After asking how things had gone since my surgery, she began explaining how the catheter removal would proceed. Significantly, she made no reference to the pathology report, which indicated to me it wasn't yet available. We had been warned this was a possibility, in which case we would receive a follow-up phone call after the catheter removal. Part of me was grateful to kick that can down the road a stretch. For now, I was happy to focus on being free of the rubber tube in my trousers. I asked Shannon what I should expect when the catheter was removed and whether it was painful. I felt a bit whiny to ask, but what the hell. There had been enough unpleasant surprises in my cancer road trip that I was disinclined to hold my tongue.

"Not painful at all," she assured me as she slipped on a pair of blue gloves. "It might feel a little weird, but it goes fast."

The Foley catheter is an ingenious device kept in place by means of an inflatable balloon on the bladder-end of the rubber tube. When filled with sterile water, the balloon secures the catheter tube snugly inside your bladder, while allowing urine to flow down the tube, by means of gravity, into the bag. Consequently, before removing the apparatus, Shannon first emptied the balloon inside me by applying a syringe to a valve on the catheter line, after which she unstrapped the bag from my leg. This next-to-final step accomplished, she took hold of the tube and said, "Okay, take a big breath."

I did, perhaps a bit dramatically.

I hoped she didn't see the white-knuckled grip I had on the side of the examination table.

"Now exhale."

As I breathed out, I felt a slight tugging inside my lower abdomen and the tube sliding painlessly through my urethra. And that was it. No muss no fuss. Shannon tossed the dishonored Mr. Foley into a plastic tub and turned to her next task. I rolled my eyes upward and breathed a sigh of relief.

Because the catheter tube runs through your johnson, down your urethra, and into your bladder, it's a bad idea to have an unsecured catheter bag swinging from your private parts like a pendulum on a cuckoo clock. For that reason, they had applied to my upper thigh a plastic clip that held the line safely in place, even when I had to change the position of the bag itself. Removing that clip took some doing, it turns out, as the manufacturer used some equivalent of Super Glue to ensure satisfactory adhesion. Shannon used a gauze square and liberal applications of alcohol to coax the stubborn adhesive to surrender its grip. Some ugly grimaces and several hundred lost leg hairs later, and the clip was off, leaving an angry-looking butterfly-shaped patch of red skin in its place.

This final, sacramental act of unshackling accomplished, I stood looking down at my naked body. No tubes. No bloated bag of urine on my calf. No clip. Just me. Images of William Wallace thundered into my consciousness, his face striped in blue war paint, his eyes alight with Scottish fervor. Deep inside me, on the rolling green field of my masculine identity, Braveheart was galloping back and forth, screaming "Freedom!" And I was digging it big-time. I was a man again.

Then Shannon handed me a pair of diapers.

They were big and bulky and crunchy feeling in my hands. Elastic around the waist and leg openings made the material bunch up like a girl's ruffly petticoat. Crestfallen, I looked at the pants I had brought to wear and wondered how I could stuff this billowy white mess into my slim-cut Banana Republic jeans. This was accomplished with considerable tucking, it turns out— but I made it work. The diapers felt strange and bulky but they were, thankfully, unnoticeable from the outside. At least that's what Barbara told me.

As I zipped up my trousers, Shannon unceremoniously dug a folded sheet of paper from the pocket of her lab coat, saying, "I've also got your pathology report, which I can go over now."

Well, that was unexpected.

A crackle of nervous energy passed between me and Barbara, though I didn't catch her eye which was fixed on Shannon. I sat back down on the examination table, the diapers crunching inside my jeans. As if on cue, my heart started pounding and blood rushed in my ears. It occurred to me that Shannon had the pathology results in her pocket all along—that she had consciously deferred sharing this news until the end of our meeting. I later concluded that Sloan Kettering staff, who deliver life-changing news almost daily, must carefully orchestrate these sensitive moments: Remove the catheter first so everyone is more relaxed, then transition to the big news in a matter-of-fact way. Don't let anxiety build. Keep it breezy. It made perfect sense, of course, but I never saw it coming. Shannon scanned the document and began casually, as if she hadn't reviewed it beforehand. "Let's see . . . " she trailed off. More choreography, I mused.

"First, your Gleason score was upgraded slightly from a three-plus-four to a four-plus-three."

A bad seven, I thought. *Not a good start.*

"Does that mean it was a more aggressive cancer?" I asked.

"It means it's good we got it out of there," she replied diplomatically.

She paused briefly as she scanned the document. The interval couldn't have been more than a second or two, but I felt like I was dangling from a rope, with Barbara and Shannon standing several feet below me. It became clear that, for all my intellectual acceptance of a possible second round of treatment, I remained terrified of the prospect.

"Your surgical margins were clear, though, which is *really* good."

Another pause.

"Seminal vesicles and bladder neck were clear."

More scanning the page.

"And your lymph nodes were clear, too." Then she smiled and looked up. "So this is a very good pathology report. I think Dr. Touijer will like this one." She added, parenthetically, "I've seen his face when he read reports he doesn't like, and I know this one will make him happy."

With that, someone pulled a plug from the examination room and all the air pressure that had suddenly built up escaped in a silent woosh, leaving Barbara and me at once deflated and ebullient. Except for the higher Gleason number, Shannon had checked all the good boxes.

"Will there be any follow-up treatment?" I asked hesitantly.

"Nope. We'll take a PSA in six weeks and, assuming it's okay, you'll have it checked every six months from here on out." She smiled, folded up the pathology report, and returned it to her pocket.

After that, she explained the logistics for the remainder of our visit. We were to stay within a few blocks of Sloan Kettering until I had my first urination, at which point I was to call Shannon and report the results. If all went well, we were free to head back to Saratoga. If, however, I experienced excruciating pain in my lower abdomen—pain that doubled me over, she elaborated—I was to let her know right away and come back to the office.

No shit, I'll let you know, I thought.

Alarmed, Barbara asked what that kind of pain meant.

Shannon had a way of sharing frightening information in a disarming way—a useful talent for a nurse at a cancer center, by the way—and explained that it meant there was a leak where my urethra had been surgically detached from the bladder and sutured back into place after prostate removal. This sounded like a horrible predicament, involving more surgery and recovery, but Shannon assured us that "It's easy to fix. It just means we put the catheter back in for another week to let it finish healing. But that's very rare. I'm sure it'll go fine." With that encouragement and some last-minute details about anticipated urinary issues, we were free to go have lunch and await my first urination as a catheter-free man with clear surgical margins.

As we left the Sidney Kimmel Center for Urologic and Prostate Cancers, I quickly texted Mattie about the pathology report, using lots of rainbow and sunshine emojis. Within seconds she replied, "BEST NEWS EVER!!!!!"

That pretty much summed it up for me.

One of the more interesting things I learned about myself when I was sick was how my mind and body responded to major disclosive milestones, these revelations of life-changing information. Because I struggled with anxiety, all such moments were replete with the turbulence of a thudding heart, shallow breathing, and a feelings of doom. To some degree, I was able to manage those physical symptoms, though never entirely eliminate them, with deep-breathing exercises and coping strategies I'd been taught in therapy. As a result of this primitive fight-or-flight response run amok, my mind was forced to function in a storm of emotion, like a commuter fumbling with a broken umbrella in a sudden downpour. My memory would refer back to articles I had read, important checklists, previous conversations—all the while sorting through the relative positives and negatives of the news I received. My mind's processing power was never strong or clear in these moments, but having Barbara there taking notes and asking questions largely addressed this deficiency. Because my physical response was so tied to anxiety, I often experienced the most comprehensive reaction to news well after my cognition had completed its assessment and passed along its conclusions to my anguished monkey brain. At that point, by means of some miracle of blood chemistry, my body would finally respond.

In this instance, that reaction took place about thirty minutes later when Barbara and I were walking around the Upper East Side looking for a lunch restaurant. I was adjusting to the feeling of wearing jeans again and the simplicity and nakedness of my unfettered private parts inside my paper diapers. The combination of my liberation from the catheter and the good pathology report began to sink into my body like rainwater and, as it did, my legs grew strangely shaky. It was an unexpected sensation, as if my body, borne down by a terrible burden, was only now feeling its weariness—or as if freedom from dread were itself a heavy load. So up Second Avenue I wobbled unsteadily but cheerfully, looking for a place to eat and, I presumed, to take my first piss without the Foley.

A short while later, we were sitting in a nearby Le Pain Quotidien restaurant drinking iced tea and eating sandwiches. Midway through lunch, nature called with slightly more urgency than usual. Apprehensive but eager to see how my rebuilt plumbing would function, I excused myself and headed to the men's room. Barbara gave me a significant look and wished me well. All things considered, it was a non-event. Shannon warned me that, for a while, it would feel "weird" when I urinated, and so it did. Overall my urinary system felt weak and uncertain, and it stung slightly to evacuate. But there in the LPQ men's room, I had an uneventful, if slightly dribbly and uncomfortable, urination. Feeling exultant, I washed my hands and stepped out of the restroom into the expectant gaze of my wife sitting some 30 feet across the restaurant. She raised her eyebrows inquiringly.

I gave her a thumbs-up as I approached the table.

After we left the restaurant, I called Touijer's office to let them know of my success. The receptionist's voice made her sound like an 18-year-old.

"Hi, this is Jim Hill. I'm calling because Shannon wanted me to report when I had my first urination after having my catheter out," I said somewhat uncertainly. "Everything, uh, went fine."

"Oh, that's excellent!" she responded.

I was momentarily back in preschool telling the teacher I had a good potty.

"You'll let Shannon know?"

"Of course. Have a great drive back!"

As Barbara and I strolled around Manhattan, the gray February sky gave way to brilliant winter sunshine and our shadows stretched out before us on the sidewalk. I made an offhand remark about the cosmic author's attempt at pathetic fallacy, a poetic practice of attributing human emotional responses to nature. Appreciating the literary reference, Barbara laughed heartily, more out of relief than amusement. The fact is, everywhere I turned, I was looking for signs that the universe acknowledged my good news. Other than the spectacular weather, though, New York City was its usual distracted self: A taxi driver honked maniacally at a FedEx truck; two Orthodox

Jewish men stood talking outside a Duane Reade; a man in dreadlocks and an Obama T-shirt was dragged along by five dogs on a tangle of leashes. Looking down from his desk, that cosmic author couldn't have missed the two middle-aged pedestrians moving purposefully along 68th Street. The woman, her blonde hair pulled back behind her head, wore dark sunglasses and walked with her face tilted upwards into the glow of the sun. The man, also in sunglasses, looked content just to walk, as if it were as novel to him as stepping among starfish scattered on an early-morning beach.

At that point, I still had five or six weeks of recovery ahead of me. I was prohibited from vigorous exercise or lifting anything heavier than ten pounds. With my catheter out and my bladder temporarily shrunken from being so under-burdened, I was warned against drinking too many fluids (a modification to my post-operative instructions to drink as much as I could manage), particularly alcohol and caffeine. I was also issued a daily, low-dose prescription for Sildenafil, the generic form of Viagra, the purpose of which was to keep the blood supply wide open to my privates so I would return to previous potency as quickly as possible. Up until this point, I had taken only a passing interest in the subject of erections, not wanting to contemplate what an inadvertent hard-on might feel like with a catheter in. But now that I was looking ahead to my continued recovery, the issue of sexual functioning came into sharper focus. My instructions said to begin taking 20 mg of Sildenafil every night before bed. Then, after a week or two, I was to take a "challenge dose" of 100 mg and record the results. The ideal outcome, I surmised, was a serviceable erection, though I was warned not to expect too much so soon after surgery, especially considering that my left nerve bundle had been affected, a reality that was underscored by a large expanse of numb skin on my upper left thigh. I had noticed that, while my brain was just as likely to experience arousal, the companion in my underwear seemed disengaged, like a sulky teenager refusing to dance at prom. To be honest, though, I wasn't concerned. I'd been warned how long recovery of potency could take; and I was more focused on getting back my fitness and regaining normal urinary functioning.

As for the standard-issue diapers I wore on the way home from Sloan Kettering, those went into the trash can as soon as I was in the house. Instead, I opted for an unobtrusive absorbent pad I could wear inside my boxer briefs (a new style of underwear I adopted as a result of the catheter, and which became my go-to option in the months after surgery). It quickly became clear that any urinary issues I had were limited to stress incontinence—the occasional drop or two that escaped when I sneezed or stood up abruptly. I was delighted to find I could get through an entire day with a single pad, and even then with only a few errant drops here and there. This was highly encouraging and soon led to my experimenting with social outings and trips to the Y. I was also advised to resume my Kegel exercises, now that the catheter was out. Before surgery, I had grown accomplished at invisible Kegel workouts, doing sets throughout the day whenever it occurred to me. Now I got back into the habit, noticing, however, that my pelvic floor muscles were substantially weaker and that an intense set or two could quickly tire them out. So I got used to emptying my bladder before I did Kegel exercises to make sure the muscular exhaustion didn't result in accidental drops between reps.

Increasingly confident I could keep my trousers dry, I resumed going to the Y, initially doing easy walks around the track, then moving to the treadmill for more vigorous stepping. This was pretty much the extent of my exercise for the first two weeks. Later, as I felt my strength returning—but against Barbara's admonitions—I undertook an experimental workout with five-pound dumbbells, technically staying under my ten-pound weight restriction, though aware Shannon might not entirely approve. Overall, it went pretty well, the weights feeling hardly as heavy as a half-gallon of milk. I figured I'd try one weight workout each week during my recovery—just enough to keep my muscles from withering entirely. Some days later, I decided to try adding dumbbell bench presses to my routine. So, taking a seat on a bench with my tiny weights in hand, I eased myself carefully on to my back. I did a light set of fifteen reps and when I tried to sit up afterwards . . . couldn't do it. Getting upright, I realized with consternation, required far too much involvement of my tender and depleted core muscles. Humbled by my overzealousness, I lay there for a moment considering how to get off the bench without looking like an upended tortoise on a desert road. After a moment of planning disguised as a rest between sets, I carefully rolled on to my side, pushed myself up on an elbow, and slid off the bench. It wasn't a high point in my recovery, but it did remind me not to rush the whole exercise thing. Nonetheless, I continued with my walking regimen and weekly, ultra-light weight training. As I regained some strength, I also got more active around the house, doing little chores and, after two or three weeks, even vacuuming. It felt good to be productive again, even though my healing body frequently reminded me to back off certain activities. Often, I would find myself so exhausted by a flurry of housework that I'd take a short nap to recover my strength.

With confidence in my body came a willingness to get more social, so Barbara and I arranged a dinner out with two of her colleagues from Skidmore College. On the whole, the evening went fine. We chose a new restaurant called the Blue Hen where none of us had been yet, and, because this was our first night out since my surgery, we were all feeling jubilant. I was aware that alcohol made my bladder control a little less reliable than usual, but I couldn't resist the temptation to order a cocktail. Aside from an extra trip to the men's room to prevent a full bladder from overburdening my modified plumbing, I didn't have any trouble. I did find myself glancing down at my crotch periodically to make sure there wasn't a wet spot somewhere (there wasn't). Aside from that mild paranoia, the night was a big success, so I crossed out another item on the checklist of recovery.

By that time we had bid farewell to February, historically one of my least favorite months (my mother died in February and my family came to regard it as the bad luck month) and moved into early March, with the promise of spring distantly in view. My recovery seemed to be proceeding expeditiously. I had only minor stress incontinence and used a single absorbent pad each day. I was walking at least 10,000 steps every day and experimenting with light weights once a week. And I was taking my 20 mg of Sildenafil as prescribed, with plans to attempt a "challenge dose" in the near future. Seeing how well things were going, we had decided to pursue a spring vacation we originally planned in the fall before my surgery. Barbara's and Mattie's spring vacations aligned nicely, so we had scheduled to fly to our family vacation home in Aspen, Colorado, for a week of relaxation for the parents, and skiing lessons for Mattie. Our flight left the morning of Sunday, March 11. Before our departure, I found myself daydreaming about reading all day by a fireplace stacked high with pine logs, watching the snow fall, and letting my body just heal. Mattie and Barbara were likewise ebullient, and as our departure drew near, we printed travel documents, extracted luggage from the linen closet, and started to pack.

These hopeful moments are often when the cosmic author, desirous of an entertaining plot twist, turns his attention from pathetic fallacy to irony.

9

FIRE IN THE HOLE

"THE CONFIRM NUMBER IS VY7LHC," Barbara said to a tinny voice on her cell phone.

I sat nearby, halfway paying attention as if from the other side of a wall.

"Yes, leaving tomorrow morning ... from Albany to Denver."

Barbara looked over at me as she listened to the Southwest Airlines agent. She was still wearing her tennis clothes from her aborted game that morning, her purse settled hurriedly at the foot of her chair. Mattie stood protectively by Barbara's side, listening to the conversation and scanning her surroundings suspiciously.

"I'm actually calling from the emergency room now," she continued. "My husband won't be able to make the trip for medical reasons, so we need to cancel."

I looked at Mattie to see how this whole thing was registering with her. She seemed stalwart, but I knew she was shell-shocked by the morning's events. Still, she had handled the whole thing courageously. Barbara jotted some notes on a pad of paper, thanked the agent, and set down her phone. "We should be all set," she said without emotion. "They'll process the outbound refund today. The return flights could take up to thirty days. They were very nice."

I pursed my lips slightly. My eyes turned downward to the wristband on my arm with my name and birthdate printed next to a barcode.

A moment later the door opened and the emergency room physician, Dr. D, strode in with a sheet of paper clutched in his hand. Barbara leaned over and dropped her phone and notepad into her purse. Mattie crossed her arms and leaned back against the wall, shooting poisonous looks at our visitor.

Dr. D glanced around the room, missing the obvious signs of hostility, and began: "I just talked to your doctor from Sloan Kettering and he doesn't think you'll need a cystogram—just the MRI."

Barbara's eyes lit up momentarily. "You talked to Dr. Touijer?"

"Yes. He called a few minutes ago."

"Wow," she mused out loud, "on a Saturday."

Unimpressed, Dr. D continued with his announcement. "The MRI didn't show any kind of tear. Your doctor thinks you probably just had a bladder spasm."

A bladder spasm sounded fairly harmless and I asked, incredulously, if such a condition could cause the kind of pain I experienced.

"They can be pretty bad," said Dr. D. Then he paused a minute and looked back over the MRI results, adding ominously, "This says that you have ascites around your liver and lower abdomen."

"What are ascites?" I asked, envisioning some kind of nasty parasite.

"It's fluid in your abdomen." Then, before I could say another word, he added, "Are you a heavy drinker?"

Stunned, I assured him that I was not a heavy drinker and, with growing irritation, asked why this mattered.

"Ascites are often a result of cirrhosis of the liver," he responded, oblivious to my astonishment.

"No," Barbara added with finality, her own anger mounting. She shot an exasperated look at me as if to say, *who is this clown?*

Undeterred, Dr. D moved on with all the deftness of a three-legged elephant. "Did they tell you," he continued, "that your cancer had spread?"

Our little family of three was good at traveling together. After taking so many international and domestic trips, we had developed good routines and divisions of labor that helped us pack efficiently and arrive at the airport on time. Each of us took pride in packing lightly and getting through vacations with only small carry-on bags. I used to brag that we took a ten-day safari in Tanzania with only three bags among us (not counting my massive new camera case bought just for the occasion). The morning before we were to depart for Colorado, I logged on to Southwest.com to print our boarding passes. Mattie and Barbara, meanwhile, assembled stacks of clothing by their black roller bags. At 9:30, we took a break to go to the Y where Barbara took a Zumba class and Mattie and I did a light workout. Knowing I'd be taking it easy in Aspen, I decided to do one of my light dumbbell sessions that morning. Mattie joined me, intrigued by my claims that I could work my muscles with only five-pound weights and lots of reps.

After the Y, we returned home where I resumed packing. Barbara changed clothes and left to meet a friend for a final set of tennis before our trip. Mattie, who had arrived home from Barnard the day before, went downstairs to call a friend. A few minutes into packing, I had to go to the bathroom, which by this time had become almost entirely normal again. Now a full month after my surgery, I was hoping to dispense with absorbent pads in my shorts in the near future. As I finished my business and zipped up my pants, I felt a warm cramping in my abdomen. Thinking it must be an onset of gas, I cursed the hefty bowl of raisin bran I ate for breakfast. Within seconds, however, the localized cramp intensified, spreading rapidly through my entire midsection. *This was some fierce gas*, I thought.

Grimacing, I headed back to the bedroom where I had been packing, the pain growing worse with every step. I decided to get on the bed and into the "plow" position, which had worked in the past to relieve gas cramps. As I lifted my legs up on the bed, though, the pain made an all-out assault, crushing my midsection in a fiery vise-grip unlike anything I'd ever experienced. I let out a groan, rolling onto my side to find a position that could ease the agony. Nothing helped. The pain intensified with my every feeble attempt to defuse it. Within a minute or two, I was completely immobilized, neither able to speak nor form coherent thoughts. There, on the rumpled bed strewn with clothes for my trip, I was frozen on all fours, sweating and gasping for air as the pain bore down on me, my head hanging hopelessly between my arms. Realizing I was in real trouble, I called downstairs to Mattie. The sound of my voice was distant and unfamiliar and, when I described it later that day to Barbara, I likened it to my father's voice when he lay confused and dying from pancreatic cancer. It was an aural expression of unremitting desperation—weak and plaintive as if from someone who'd fallen into a deep crevasse and could neither relieve his pain nor orient himself in the fathomless dark. Never before have I experienced such dissociation, such physical dislocation, from myself.

In a moment Mattie was in the bedroom, desperately trying to understand what was happening. She told me later she thought I was dying of a heart attack. It must have looked that way: I was sweating heavily and my breathing was a slow, rhythmic gasping, like a woman in labor sucking in air as a bulwark against the agony.

"Call 911," I groaned, aware I might black out.

"What do I tell them? Oh my god!" She was on the verge of sobbing, but I couldn't say anything to reassure her.

Eventually, between searing knife plunges in my lower abdomen, I managed to get out, "Tell them . . . I had prostate surgery . . . think it's a tear where my urethra . . . was cut from the bladder . . . " Every word was an agony.

In a few seconds, Mattie had a 911 operator on the phone and, at her request, put me on speaker. The operator began asking about the pain and my recent medical history. She was very calm. I was not.

I remember screaming at her to *get me a fucking ambulance and stop asking me fucking stupid questions.*

Mattie, now inflamed by my mania, uncharacteristically joined in, screaming something about hurrying the fuck up.

My eyes were closed, my jaw clamped shut.

An eternity later, I heard Mattie downstairs letting someone in the front door, then heavy footsteps on the wooden stairs.

Several bodies entered the bedroom with a gust of cool air, though I did not, could not, look up to acknowledge them.

A male voice to the left of me asked about my cancer. What stage was it? How bad was the pain? Scale of one to 10.

"SEVENTY FIVE," I screamed from the roiling pool of magma in my midsection.

He asked me to roll over on my side so they could prepare an IV.

NO FUCKING WAY.

You can do it. Come on. Easy. There you go.

Cold alcohol swab on my skin. A needle poke.

Then I was being moved into a strange sedan chair, strapped in, and heaved down our narrow wooden stairs. My eyes opened briefly to see three men guiding me down the steps as the chair swayed from side to side. Outside the house, I was lifted from the chair on to a stretcher and loaded into the ambulance. That's when I felt the drugs kick in, like a hot, shimmering wave that began in my head and radiated downward into my seized-up body. By the time the EMTs closed the ambulance door behind me, I could feel the pain in my abdomen relaxing its grip, like a grizzly bear grown tired of its dying plaything. With the agony abating, my shell-shocked consciousness reasserted itself, elbowing its way up to the front of my mind. Taking stock of my surroundings, I looked through the back window to where a heartbreaking tableau was forming in front of our house: Mattie stood tall and alone by the wrought iron gate, still in her sweats, her long blonde hair pulled back in a disheveled ponytail. Her arms were crossed against her chest and her lips were slightly parted. As Mattie watched me drive away, Barbara and her tennis partner pulled up in front of the house. The car door swung open and Barbara launched from the car with her tennis racket in hand. She rushed to Mattie's side and embraced her protectively, her gaze moving desperately from the ambulance to her bleary-eyed daughter.

All I could think about as my wife and daughter receded into the distance was that I had just blown up their spring break.

By the time we reached the hospital, I was loopy from the morphine I'd been given at the house. I mentioned to the EMT that my nose itched a lot, which, he explained, is a side effect of opioid painkillers. I realized with a glimmer of hope that my head must be clearing to have noticed something so insignificant. Somewhere around the intersection of Church and Clinton Streets, the pain dropped from ten to a more manageable six or seven, at which point I regained my manners and thanked the EMTs for putting up with all my f-bombs and obstinance.

"No worries," one of them laughed. Then he smiled knowingly at his colleague and added, "We've heard a lot worse than that."

A few blurry minutes later, I was in an examination room being looked over by various people. Much more alert now, I was able to provide details on my recent medical history, emphasizing my theory I had experienced a leak in the urethra as a result of my prostatectomy—the phenomenon Shannon had warned us about three weeks earlier. Each time I made this assertion, however, I lost the attention of whomever I was speaking with, as though my insights were merely distracting to them.

Dr. D came by a number of times in the first hour or so. As I recall, he wore a white coat over his street clothes. His name was embroidered on his coat pocket in decorative cursive lettering, as if a proud wife had presented it to him one Christmas. He stood about six feet tall. His face was thin and unremarkable, with the skin tones of a white man who seldom steps outdoors. Lacking any notable facial architecture, he had grown a sparse beard, reminding me of a gardener who festoons a chain-link fence with honeysuckle. Slender and unmuscular, Dr. D's most prominent feature was a pronounced potbelly that had no clear relationship to the rest of his body. This unfortunate cynosure inevitably drew one's eyes to his midsection whenever he appeared. Early in my interactions with him, I concluded Dr. D was not a man with deep reserves of self-confidence. That I had surgery at Sloan Kettering and was under the care of an exotic-sounding surgeon seemed to get under his skin. In my first exchanges with the hospital room nurses, I had pleaded with them to contact Sloan Kettering. Dr. D had come to announce that he had, apparently with reluctance, complied.

"We called Sloan Kettering and I spoke to one of the fellows in their urology department," he explained with a detectable eye-roll. "He wants us to run an MRI and a cystogram to see if you have a leak at the surgical site."

This corresponded with my expectations, and I nodded in agreement.

"The nurse tells me you're retaining urine, though. She said you had about 700 cc's in your bladder when you came in."

I explained that I had consumed a lot of coffee and water that morning and had been avoiding urination since my painful episode, assuming that peeing had caused the whole thing. So it was no surprise, I continued, that I had urine in my bladder. My explanation, however, seemed to flutter past Dr. D's ears like barn swallows, disappearing into the emergency room hallway.

"We're going to need you to urinate so we can get a urine sample," he persisted.

Barbara stood up as if to launch into a diatribe, but I beat her to the punch. "I'm not going to urinate," I said emphatically. "That pain almost killed me. I think I need to get a catheter in to avoid a leak."

"We don't know you have a leak," Dr. D responded with the tone of an affronted librarian.

"There's no way I'm going to urinate."

"I've ordered an MRI," said the doctor, changing subjects slightly. "It could take a little while to get that set up. In the meantime, I'll talk to Sloan Kettering about the catheter."

About an hour later, I was taken in for an MRI and then returned to my examination room where Barbara and Mattie waited. Shortly after that, Dr. D returned and explained that he had spoken to the fellow at Sloan Kettering again who recommended putting in a catheter to take the burden off my bladder. I breathed a sigh of relief. That I was happy to be re-acquainted with the catheter was an indication of my desperation to avoid the pain of that morning. As Dr. D left the room, a short, heavyset nurse came in with a tray of materials. She was a chatty, middle-aged woman who did not inspire confidence. As she unwrapped and arranged her instruments, she explained how infrequently the emergency room staff were called upon to insert catheters. "Rest assured," she said unconvincingly, "I'm sure we'll figure it out. They trained us on all this."

I did not rest assured.

Now, I had been happily unconscious when my first Foley was inserted; I awoke to see it extending from my plumbing as if it had been there for months. And although removing the catheter was less unpleasant than I had expected, having it inserted while conscious did not sound promising at all. I was more right than wrong. Without going into unappealing detail, I'll simply say that the highlight of the procedure, which the nurse began and aborted several times in frustration, was when the struggling caregiver, catheter tube in one hand and my helpless johnson in the other, looked at Barbara and said, "Okay, this is the hard part . . . there's a place where the urethra hits the bladder and you have to kind of push on through . . . "

My eyes rolled skyward as she threaded that nasty instrument into my privates, my mind screaming execrations at the gods. Eventually, she got past whatever the "hard part" was and injected the catheter with saline to secure it in place.

"See?" she exclaimed triumphantly pointing to a stream of pale yellow working its way down the catheter tube. "You're already emptying out!" Less enthusiastic than the nurse, I lay back and let go a massive sigh.

As the nurse cleaned up, she entertained us with stories of her planned vacation to the Adirondacks and how she loved water skiing and hiking. Barbara and I listened politely, wondering why, at this particular moment, we should give a rat's ass about her vacation plans, especially after her clumsiness with the catheterization. Nonetheless, when she was done, we wished her a happy vacation and sent her on her way, forcing smiles and expressions of gratitude.

This brings us to the moment when Dr. D returned to tell me he had spoken to Touijer and that I had ascites in my abdomen. It was also when he asked, almost rhetorically, whether I'd been told that my cancer had spread.

Barbara and I hardly knew how to respond to this last question. "They never said anything about my cancer spreading," I assured him. "And my pathology report was really good."

Dr. D listened and nodded, lost in some apparent thought process. "Okay, well, ascites can indicate that the cancer has spread to other organs. But you can talk to your doctor about that. I'll give you a copy of the report to pass along." Then he appeared to brighten up, as if a cheerful thought occurred to him. "You know, I predicted we'd see some fluid in the abdomen from the surgery and, sure enough, there was some."

I didn't know if I was expected to congratulate him on this triumph. Connecting the dots, I asked if the surgery could have accounted for the ascites he referred to. "Maybe. You'll have to ask your doctor." Then he paused again and added with a slight smirk, "It's funny dealing with these big hospitals. First the fellow down there tells me to get an MRI and a cystogram. Then your doctor overrules him and says the MRI is just fine. Seems like they're not communicating too well . . ."

Ah, I thought to myself. *So this was all about medical one-upmanship*—like the plumber assessing a predecessor's soldering work with a disapproving click of his tongue. Though I understood intellectually this must occur in the medical profession as much as anywhere else, I was nonetheless stunned to see it play out in these circumstances—as if asserting one's medical credentials rightly upstaged a patient in distress. Neither Barbara nor I indulged Dr. D in this line of thought. In fact, Barbara took every opportunity to rave about Sloan Kettering and Dr. Touijer, which had minimal effect as far as I could tell.

Before long, I was cleared to return home, with instructions to contact Touijer on Monday morning. I was given a new bag of catheter supplies and a print-out on urine retention and bladder spasms and what they mean. Apparently, Dr. D and his staff weren't buying into my theory of urinary leakage caused by a tear at my surgical site. With a new catheter in place and no clarity on what had caused my pain, I headed home in a mood as black as the dregs in my coffee cup.

The following Monday morning, I was lying awake in bed, debating whether to get up and begin the process of emptying my catheter bag, showering, and changing into my day bag. I could hear Barbara making her morning tea in the kitchen downstairs. As I lay there feeling sorry for myself and wondering how I took such a massive step backwards, my phone rang.

The caller ID read "Touijer's Office." Expecting Shannon to be on the line, I was surprised to hear a French accent: "Hello, James, it's Dr. Touijer. I heard you had a rough weekend." I was relieved to speak to him and launched into all the gory details of my weekend and aborted spring break. Feeling guilty, I asked if perhaps my return to exercise might have resulted in a torn suture. He laughed and chided, "Well, I'm not going to blame you for what happened." After a brief pause he added, "It's about a month after your surgery, so it would be very unusual for that to have occurred. If it was a leak, it most likely happened when you experienced the pain—when you urinated."

We discussed the possibility of a bladder spasm, which Touijer still felt could have been the cause, adding that my bladder may have become overburdened by retained urine, leading to a nasty spasm. "Really bad bladder spasms can feel like labor pains," he explained. "So, yeah, they can really hurt."

"Wow," I mused, thinking Barbara could no longer claim that only women experience the pain of childbirth. I had a brief vision of the old Greek prophet Tiresias, who lived as a woman for seven years. *At least women get a child out of the experience,* I thought indulgently. *I just got another catheter.*

I asked Touijer about Dr. D's reference to ascites in my abdomen, a subject that had been gnawing at me all weekend. With his usual diplomacy, he indicated that, as an emergency room physician, Dr. D had probably never seen an MRI of a man recovering from prostate surgery and simply mistook normal post-surgical fluid as something more concerning. Ascites, he said, can be a symptom of cirrhosis or a malignancy in the abdomen, which would account for Dr. D's questions about my drinking habits and my cancer having spread. Neither scenario was a concern, however, Touijer assured me, and I shouldn't lose any sleep over it. In describing my conversation with Dr. D, I wasn't as gracious as Touijer in extending Dr. D the benefit of the doubt. In fact, I was still furious that, in the midst of our disastrous trip to the emergency room, we had to deal with Dr. D's jaw-dropping lack of empathy. I think I'm still angry about it.

As we wrapped up our conversation, Touijer gave me his recommendation: "I think the thing to do is have you keep the catheter in for this week. That will take the strain off your bladder and let it recover. Then you should come back in to have it removed on the 15th." Resigned to my sentence, I thanked him for being in touch and rolled out of bed to face five more days with my old nemesis.

Intense physical pain, it turns out, leaves deep grooves in one's memory. As I anticipated having my catheter removed a second time, I found myself terrified by the prospect of that first, perilous urination. If my agony had been the result of a bladder spasm, what if the bladder remained weak from another five days of catheterization and went right back into its torment? If the pain was caused by a leak of urine into my peritoneum, what if the tiny hole hadn't healed yet? I fretfully rehearsed these possibilities to myself all week as Thursday approached. Our appointment was at 10:30 AM, so once again we rose early and made the trip to the Upper East Side. The catheter removal went much the same as the first one had: Shannon emptied the bladder balloon with a syringe, unstrapped my bag, told me to take a big breath, and pulled the catheter out. No white knuckles or anything. Then she repeated the instructions she gave me the first time, asking that I stay around Sloan Kettering until I had a full urination, at which point I was to call their office to report the results. Then I could leave town a free man.

We followed Shannon's instructions to the letter and, when nature called, I ducked into a Starbucks restroom to attempt the terrifying deed. Standing at the urinal, I found my body stubbornly non-compliant with the demands of my bladder. That deep-grooved memory was resisting anything that might release a red-hot lava flow in my abdomen. With some focused deep breathing and exhortations to my urinary system, I was able first to release some reluctant drops and, eventually, an unsteady stream. As I finished, I reflexively paused at the urinal as if awaiting the onslaught of pain. When no such discomfort occurred, I gave a sigh, washed my hands, and rejoined Barbara on the sidewalk outside.

Having cleared this milestone, I called Touijer's office with the good news and, after walking around town much as we'd done the previous time, headed back to our car for the drive home. As we passed by MSK's Sidney Kimmel Center where our appointment had been, I felt the need to urinate again, so I used their lobby restroom. Attempting my second freestyle event, I was still full of apprehension, but was relieved to experience similar success. My recovery feeling complete, I settled into the passenger seat of our car and we headed out of town, chatting confidently about the resumption of my path toward normalcy. After getting past some traffic congestion on the Henry Hudson and the George Washington Bridge, Barbara steered on to the Palisades Parkway heading north, about which time I felt mother nature's beckoning yet again. As had been the case with my previous catheter removal, my bladder capacity was diminished and I was in no mood to push my luck. So Barbara pulled up at a gas station along the parkway and I headed inside.

This time, I had no trouble going at all. I zipped up, washed my hands, and headed out of the mini-mart. Barbara was filling the car with gas, and I headed across the parking lot to meet her at the pump. As I did, the familiar hot cramping bloomed inside my abdomen and, as I took a couple more steps, set in like a vise grip. Each step became more halting and I crossed my arms protectively against my lower torso. Standing at the gas pump, Barbara noticed my altered gait and what must have been a waxen expression on my face. When I got to the car, the pain was intense, though not as horrific as my first event.

"The pain is back," I groaned, as I eased myself cautiously into the passenger seat.

The next two weeks were a frustrating tautology of pain, phone consultations, and tests to determine why I had these inexplicable episodes. After my first recurrence at the gas station, the agony eased after about twenty minutes of deep breathing and sitting stock-still in the passenger seat. Barbara called Touijer's office from the car and we spoke with a urology fellow who advised that the bladder spasms may have returned but were unlikely to continue. He recommended taking Tylenol and calling back in the morning if things didn't improve. A couple hours after we arrived home in Saratoga, I found myself needing to go, as they say in pre-school, number one and number two. By this time it was early evening and dark outside.

I knew from experience that my body was unlikely to let go of its burden willingly, given the prospect of the pain returning. So, like a housewife in the old Calgon commercial, I dimmed the lights in the bathroom, lit an aromatherapy candle, and sat down to convince my body to do what must be done.

It must have taken thirty minutes. Each time I made progress with number two, I felt number one easing up the pipe, at which point my monkey brain screamed, "Oh, no you don't," and shut the whole process down. Over and over this played out until, through sheer patience and tenacity, I managed to complete the deed—with only a hint of pain. I emerged from my makeshift spa and shared my success with Barbara with cautious optimism. *Maybe this whole thing might work out after all,* I thought.

Around 10 we went to bed, exhausted from the day's ups and downs. As I fell asleep, I had new confidence that today's setback may have been an aberration. Then, at 4 AM, I awoke suddenly, my bladder full to capacity and screaming to be emptied. It occurred to me that my caution last night might have prevented me from completely emptying my bladder, leaving me with a bigger burden now. Warily, I rose from bed and headed down the dark hallway to the bathroom, feeling as distended as a pregnant woman. As I approached the bathroom, the muscles in my urinary system, in apparent anticipation of relief, relaxed slightly—at which point the familiar pain returned—but this time like a screaming hot freight train in the night, all without even a trickle of urine passing from my body. I huddled over in the middle of the hallway, caught between the desperate need to pee and the pain radiating throughout my midsection. I limped back to the bedroom where I perched myself naked on the side of the bed, sucking in deep breaths and waiting for the spell to pass. When I began to shiver, Barbara threw a blanket over my shoulders and sat watching me with concern. After a half-hour, the grizzly bear released me from its jaws once again. Exhausted, I slid under the covers, my bladder still aching to be emptied, and tried to fall asleep.

That morning, after another consultation with a fellow at Touijer's office, we headed to a nearby urgent care center in Saratoga where we explained the situation and asked that they insert yet another catheter at the request of my surgeon. My experience at the urgent care center wasn't as bad as at the local emergency room. The physician on hand was a pleasant, competent man in his early forties who seemed focused on making me as comfortable as possible. He directed his staff to put the catheter back in as quickly as possible. His staff showed less confidence in how to proceed than he did. The nurse charged with the task had to go find a catheter and later, when experiencing difficulty completing the insertion (at this point having the tube wedged halfway up inside me), asked for help from her colleagues. First, someone named Nina came in, but she felt Ron might be most helpful. Ron was occupied elsewhere at the moment, so while the first nurse held the catheter in place and tried to make small talk, Nina went looking for the man in question. I lay on the examination room table half-naked and exasperated, counting the seconds and staring at the ceiling. When he arrived, Ron assessed the situation, took the catheter tube in one hand and my traumatized penis in the other and went to work. Apparently Ron's reputation for skill with catheters had more to do with strength than technique. Where the first nurse had struggled ineffectually to finish the task, Ron wrenched my manhood like it was a tube of toothpaste, ramming the catheter so aggressively inside me I nearly passed out.

"Ahhhhh," I groaned as he flattened my penis between his fingers. You'd have thought a fellow man would empathize with the pain he was inflicting on another man's genitals. But he seemed intent only on driving that catheter tube home and returning to whatever Netflix movie he was streaming on his cell phone in the break area.

Barbara heard the entire ordeal from the other side of a curtain. I asked that she not watch the procedure, as I still hoped to retain some shred of sexual mystery for the woman I loved. I can only imagine how the drama sounded from where she sat.

"Oh, Ron! Good. I can't get the Foley past this spot here . . . "

"Here, let me try. Sometimes you just have to push past it . . . "

"Uhhhh."

"Sorry. Hang on. I'm almost there."

"Fuck . . . FUCK."

"Just a little farther. The tube can get hung up here . . . "

"There it is . . . see? Okay, give me the syringe."

After this latest episode, Touijer speculated I might have a leak after all. This wasn't sounding like bladder spasms anymore. He asked me to come see him on March 23rd in Sloan Kettering's Westchester facility in West Harrison, New York, north of the City, where they would give me a cystogram—an MRI of my bladder filled to capacity with liquid contrast medium—to determine if any such leak existed. In the meantime, I was facing another seven days with the Foley. Though the week that transpired wasn't as eventful as the previous few days, it did bring some disconcerting new developments. The day after my date with Nina and Ron, I noticed the liquid in my catheter bag was the color of rosé wine, indicating there was bleeding in my urinary tract. I reported this to Shannon who wasn't alarmed but asked that I keep her apprised of any other changes. A day later, as I attempted the always-awkward process of having a bowel movement with a catheter in place, I noticed bloody urine running down the outside of the catheter tube, and dripping into the toilet. This was new. Within seconds of the bloody drops appearing, the familiar pain made its appearance, at which point my system shut down and all hope of a bowel movement ended. Frustration and despair clouded my mind as I sat on the toilet clutching my midsection. So I had a catheter in and still had the pain. Now what?

Another call to Shannon.

She assured me that some leakage from around the catheter wasn't unusual during a bowel movement, especially if one "pushes hard." As for the blood, she explained, that was also fairly normal and suggested that perhaps the reinsertion of the catheter had beat me up a little inside.

I needed no convincing of that likelihood.

But what about the return of the pain, I asked? How could that happen with the catheter in?

She explained that if I had even a tiny leak, a few drops of urine that didn't pass through the catheter but went by, shall we say, the conventional route, could have caused the pain.

Urine is highly acidic and the tiniest amount of it leaking into the peritoneum was likely to cause significant discomfort. However, any such leak would be detected by the cystogram I had scheduled for the 23rd. All this was reassuring, though it introduced the startling new possibility that each time I had a bowel movement, I might also have the pain. This revelation gave an entirely new dimension to my bathroom experiences for the remainder of the week: My Pavlovian subconscious was more terrified of the pain than it was motivated to relieve itself. The result was multiple unproductive trips to the restroom, during which I tried every conceivable position to minimize leakage and maximize potential for a successful "outcome." I used the stool softener I had been prescribed after surgery. I drank prune juice and ate bran flakes. I elevated my feet on a cardboard box. Anything to make number two's go so smoothly they didn't induce a leak.

It would be an understatement to say that these weeks of being in and out of emergency rooms and urgent care centers, of being catheterized and re-catheterized, of cajoling my shell-shocked body to comply with my simplest wishes, were hard on my middle-aged male self-esteem. Before commencing my hike along the prostate cancer trail, I was mortified even to drop my trousers, turn my head, and cough for a hernia check. Since the disclosure that my previously healthy prostate was hiding a dark secret, I had undergone every indignity I could imagine, the net effect of which was that each devolution of my male pride brought a loss in perspective on how privacy, sexuality, even masculine confidence felt. Like a hiker who had tumbled down a ravine and lay bleeding on a bed of cacti, I looked up at the slope from which I'd fallen with mixed emotions: frustration that I fell, and relief that the ravine wasn't a cliff. I didn't know if I should be grateful to have my masculine pride so humbled, or to be bitter that so little of it remained. Any optimism I managed that week arose from anticipation of the next opportunity for relief from my immediate circumstances. And at this juncture, the next such opportunity was on Friday March 23rd, at Sloan Kettering's Westchester facility. There I would have the integrity of my urinary system scanned for leaks and, assuming none existed, have my catheter removed for a third time. I didn't allow myself to think "third time's a charm." Mostly, I just sent encouraging thoughts to the cells hard at work repairing the leak. We were all on the clock at that point: Finish the job by Friday or I was looking at more prison time.

10

REPRIEVE

IT'S A HELL OF A GIG being the partner of a cancer patient.

Often, I tried to imagine myself in Barbara's position, and I always decided that her role in our family drama was tougher than mine. Though I was the recipient of the cancer diagnosis, I had also been conferred a license to pity myself, brood darkly for hours, show irritation at the slightest provocation, and generally be poor company for long stretches. Barbara, in contrast, suffered right alongside me but, by some unspoken cultural convention, felt disallowed from expressing the same emotional highs and lows. Undoubtedly, much of our divergent behavior arose from our different personalities. I have always been given to saturnine brooding, finding darkness even in a context most would see as encouraging. As a teenager I wrote one bad poem after another, all contemplating sorrow, loss, and death, all abundant with images of crepuscular skies, dripping caverns, and endless fields of white poppies. Though I think of myself as fundamentally optimistic, my personal brand of optimism is tinged with a dour humorlessness. My outlook on life sounded something like a page from Tolkien: You may well arrive at your destination, but most of the road will be through nasty places like Mirkwood and Moria, with few opportunities to re-provision in sunny Rivendell. When Barbara met me in Oxford, where literary comparisons were the order of the day, she quickly identified me as Byronic—which became a handy euphemism for my gloomy preoccupation with loss and mortality.

When I began psychotherapy in late 2016, my psychotherapist Ranjit had encouraged me to explore this side of myself, even asking me to write accounts of my childhood. The usual dark imagery showed up in that work as well. Before long, we were discussing the death of my mother and its impact on my 7-year-old self. We imagined the atmosphere in the Hill household in the months before my mother's death and how it must have cast a pall over our lives. We talked about how losing a figure as central as one's mother might make one terrified to part from or, God forbid, lose loved ones. As reluctant as I had been to acknowledge that trauma in one's youth permanently changes one's outlook in life, I couldn't deny the connection. And while these revelations didn't make me a more cheerful person *per se,* they helped me understand the etiology of my unique disposition. Of course, the whole reason I turned to Ranjit was to address the anxiety that had reared up so fiercely when I left my career. Later, when I received my cancer diagnosis, I remarked sarcastically to Barbara that I couldn't imagine a better affliction for someone with anxiety. Here I was, an anxious (it turned out) middle-aged man who was preoccupied with aging, loss, and mortality, merging on to the Cancer Highway with its unreliable road signs, detours, and cliffside bends without guardrails.

The person riding beside me on this unplanned trip couldn't have been selected more strategically, though, in truth, it was blind luck. Like me, Barbara Black was the youngest of five children, but she grew up in a small town in Pennsylvania Amish country where her father was the president of the local bank and her mother was an English professor at a liberal arts college. Brought up in the Anabaptist Church of the Brethren, Barbara remembered going to Sunday services that included ritually washing the calloused, yellow feet of elderly ladies who wore stockings, rubber-snap garters, and orthopedic shoes. Every Easter, the choir delivered an enthusiastic rendition of "Up From the Grave He Arose," and on Sundays the pastor spent more time giving updates on church missions to Uganda than upbraiding sinners. In her hometown of Elizabethtown, Pennsylvania, Barbara's parents and grandparents were like local aristocracy, and the five Black children saw themselves as upholding a reputation of gentility and elegance. As the youngest, Barbara idolized her siblings, adopting many of their intellectual and musical interests. Her brother Merle, a brilliant student, studied German intellectual history at the University of Chicago, and Barbara honored him by immersing herself in Kant, Nietzsche, and Hegel. Her oldest sister Phyllis earned her PhD in English Literature at West Virginia University and eventually married Russ MacDonald, one of her professors there. Russ and Phyllis, and Barbara's mother, Louise, who taught at Elizabethtown College, influenced her eventual choice of English Literature as a focus, to which she switched after a brief dalliance with a philosophy major. Meanwhile, her father Merle, a taciturn, dignified, self-made man of humble Appalachian roots, instilled in her an unshakeable sense of honor and a fierce, leonine loyalty.

In high school Barbara played the viola, danced ballet and jazz, and led the E-town marching band as its drum major—not the baton-tossing majorette, she would point out, but the high-stepping, mace-wielding martinet who leads the band across the field in perfect cadence. She was a star student in her rural high school; and Bryn Mawr College, a challenging women's liberal arts institution on Philadelphia's Main Line, welcomed her to its freshman class in 1980. There, she joined a string quartet, eventually burning herself out on too many wedding-day performances of *Eine Kleine Nachtmusik*. She grew to love Motown, Al Jarreau, and the B52s; had a couple of serious boyfriends; celebrated Lantern Night every fall; and danced around the Maypole on Merion Green every spring. After four years, she graduated *magna cum laude*, emerging from Bryn Mawr an ardent feminist, a scholar passionately committed to the humanities, and a top prospect for graduate school. This was a no-drama achiever, a woman who loved her work and whose dedication to her pursuits dutifully repaid her with accolades—as though the clockwork universe functioned properly and divine justice reigned supreme.

At the University of Virginia, Barbara focused on Victorian literature and the intimidating (at least to me) works of Eliot, Ruskin, Browning, Tennyson, and Dickens. After an arduous course of study, she wrote her dissertation on an iconic nineteenth-century English civic institution, the museum. She completed her degree in 1991, and on a beautiful May morning in Charlottesville strode up to the dais in her gown and mortarboard to receive her diploma and, to her astonishment, the Shannon Award, given to the top student in the Graduate School of Arts and Sciences.

Later that year, Elizabethtown's *enfant terrible* and I moved to Saratoga Springs, got married, and launched our more-or-less adult lives.

In 1997 we learned that Barbara was pregnant with our daughter Madeleine, who made her appearance at 1:36 AM on a cold February night in 1998. Barbara's identity at that point became bifurcated, as happens to so many women who split time between career and family. Shepherding a new human being from infancy to adulthood while teaching, publishing, and serving on countless committees, she somehow managed to get it all done with a kind of quiet determination I could only wonder at. Whenever things got tough for us, Barbara would exclaim "*Ataraxia*, Babe!" invoking the Greek word for "equanimity" I once used to characterize her preternatural calm. In the years since UVa, Barbara has published two books (with a third completed and awaiting publication) and countless articles, earned tenure, served as the reviews editor of a literary journal, won Skidmore's distinguished teaching award, and been promoted to full professor.

Friends of ours have quipped that, when I talk about Barbara, I sound like her public relations agency. It's true that I'm deeply impressed by my own spouse—maybe even a little in awe. Barbara would be quick to point out that she has seen her share of disappointment and humiliation, has suffered at the hands of what she calls the "cosmic joker," the divine troublemaker who takes a dark delight in irony. His panoptic view of simultaneous, interconnected realities makes a mockery of our blinkered human perspective, like the automobile accident unfolding in Grant Wood's "Death on Ridge Road." In that painting, a sleek black car careens up a winding hillside road, unaware of a red truck, its front tires turned and slightly airborne, approaching from the hill's other side. It is an image of imminent death, of disaster suspended in perpetuity. Neither driver is aware of the calamity about to occur; yet the casual viewer of the artwork beholds the entire scene with a sense of omniscient helplessness. This is the perspective of the cosmic joker, though he is far from helpless, his dark machinations having guided these two vehicles to their fateful meeting.

Because of the cosmic joker, Barbara never quite trusts good fortune, always expecting some ironic twist to a story before the ending arrives. It's true that she took her knocks in graduate school when, for example, the cantankerous Victorian scholar Cecil Lang excoriated her for her Germanic prose style. Or when her full-ride scholarship was temporarily scaled back in an apparent display of institutional disappointment. Along the way in life, she lost both her parents to protracted battles with Parkinson's disease, had her share of serious health scares, and like me, struggles with the insults of middle age. For all her glossy exterior and sunny disposition, she is a brilliant, complex, emotional woman on whose sensibility life has deeply inscribed, yes, happiness and success, but also loss, sadness, frustration, and failure.

For those reasons, Barbara has her own touch of the sardonic—and that may be where our two world views intersect the most. Certainly that was the case during my cancer diagnosis and treatment, when every new disclosure seemed to bring a gift from the cosmic troublemaker. Though we were both essentially hopeful, even optimistic, about the outcome, neither one of us *expected* much good news along the way. Barbara referred to that outlook as "defensive pessimism," a clinical concept she chanced upon in her reading, claiming she inherited the proclivity from her father who, though he was a successful bank president, always felt one step away from "the poor house." The "defensive" aspect of that attitude, I think, helped us weather the storms of diagnosis, treatment, and what in March of 2018 felt like constant setbacks.

As available as Barbara tended to be for my various trips

to Sloan Kettering, the 23rd of March presented a scheduling problem. All that year she had been working with a colleague in the Classics department to launch a Center for Humanistic Inquiry at Skidmore, which would debut with a symposium where members of the faculty could gather to present their work and celebrate the abiding importance of the Humanities. It was a labor of love for her, and the event began the same day I was scheduled for my cystogram at the MSK West Harrison facility. We quickly concluded there was no way Barbara could miss this first CHI event, so after some research, I arranged for a town car to take me to my appointment. As it turns out, Barbara's brother Merle, who taught history at a private school in Cincinnati, delighted her by announcing that he and his wife, Sue, were flying out to attend the symposium. It was a big couple of days for Barbara and, while I had planned to attend the entire event as well, I was prevented from doing so by the reappearance of my old companion, the Foley catheter.

On Thursday evening, Merle and Sue arrived in Saratoga, and at 4:30 the next morning, my town car pulled up outside our house to deliver me to Sloan Kettering for my 7:30 check-in. Feeling hopeful my catheter might be removed, I took along a pair of jeans into which I could change. I slept most of the way in the car and arrived feeling groggy, apprehensive, and in dire need of caffeine. In the lobby, I texted Barbara to let her know I'd arrived and to wish her luck with the symposium. She responded with her characteristic encouragement and a single heart emoji.

Sloan Kettering's West Harrison facility is a stunning building: modern, sleek, and spacious with huge windows and a flood of natural light. Dr. Touijer worked out of that location on certain days of the week and, given the scheduling challenges caused by my setbacks, asked that I meet him there rather than postpone our visit until he was in Manhattan again. After being checked in and shown to a dressing room, I changed into a hospital gown. After a twenty-minute wait, a young woman showed me into a room where an MRI machine and several expectant staff stood ready to plumb the mysteries of my bladder. The purpose of the cystogram was to get a clear look at what was causing my pain—specifically, whether I had sprung a leak in my urinary plumbing. The process involved using the catheter tube to fill my tank to capacity with a "contrast medium." Then, with the bladder fully distended, they take images from various angles and forward the results to a radiologist for review.

The attractive young doctor in charge explained that she would infuse contrast into my bladder until I let her know it was becoming uncomfortable.

"How uncomfortable?" I asked.

"We want the bladder as full as possible," she said with a deadpan expression. "So you should let it get pretty uncomfortable—like you have to pee *really* badly. But it won't last long."

And that's what we did. She poured fluid into my catheter tube, and I gave her updates on my escalating state of desperation. At last, when I had achieved college-freshman-at-a-kegger-with-no-bathroom-around desperation, I let her know. At that point, they loaded me into the MRI and took a series of images. Then, with merciful alacrity, they uncorked me.

Sixty minutes and one large coffee later, I met with Dr. Touijer in a spacious consultation room with upholstered chairs, a desk, and a computer. He was as nattily dressed as ever and had grown a beard. I complimented him on the new look and, rubbing the snowy stubble on my chin, noted he had no gray in his beard yet. He chuckled softly and apologized for making me wait so long after the cystogram.

"I actually checked with two radiologists on your images, so it took some extra time," Touijer began. The first radiologist didn't see anything out of order. But then he called in a favor with a radiologist friend, who examined the images as well—and found something. As he had with my first MRI images, Touijer turned the computer monitor toward me, selected the best image, and walked me through the findings. The images he showed me were incredibly detailed, like illustrations in an anatomy textbook—not the usual fuzzy black-and-white I'd come to expect. My bladder showed up as a large, pink, three-dimensional melon inside a uniformly monotone skeleton.

Touijer zoomed in on a spot at the bottom of the bladder where my urethra connected to it. He manipulated the image to one side and pointed with his pen. "See here? This little wisp?"

I nodded that I did see it. It was a tiny speck of pink outside the bladder.

"That's the leak. It's really small, which is why the first radiologist didn't see it," he said with a quiet tone of triumph in his voice. "It's nearly healed up, but I think we should leave the catheter in for another five days. You're already scheduled to come in on the 28th for your six-week PSA test, so let's use that time slot for another cystogram and, assuming everything goes well, we'll take the catheter out then."

I'll admit I was crestfallen to face another five days with Foley, but with the end so clearly in sight, I was prepared to soldier forth. "Sounds like a plan," I said as I stood to go.

As I gathered my things and headed for the door, Touijer logged out of the computer and remarked offhandedly, "You know, while you're here, let's go ahead and do your PSA test. We're close enough to six weeks now."

Damn, I thought, *I was almost out the door, too.* This was not what I wanted to hear. Ever since I received my encouraging pathology report, I regarded the six-week PSA test with dread. That's the thing with cancer: Good news only lasts until the next test result, at which point all the optimism of the previous few weeks or months can vanish with a single bad number. The March 28th appointment had been prominent on my Google calendar ever since my surgery. It would be the first assessment of my PSA levels since the December day when Dr. Z reported my number had shot up to 19.6. This test, even more than my post-surgical pathology report, could change everything. If my results showed a lingering presence of prostate-specific antigen, it meant the cancer remained somewhere inside me and that more treatment, probably radiation and perhaps even adjuvant hormone therapy, lay ahead. It also meant my odds of getting sicker, or even dying, were dramatically higher. If the results were clear, well, then fireworks and champagne toasts.

I got a little cowardly at this point and asked if running the test prematurely might give a false positive. I knew from my reading that the body needed about six weeks to flush residual PSA out of its system.

"I think it's enough time," he said. "There really shouldn't be any antigen left at this point. If there is, it probably isn't residual."

I grasped his meaning immediately and decided to discontinue this line of questioning. As Touijer bade his farewell, Shannon, who was also working at the Westchester location that day, came in to explain how the testing would go. She told me where the phlebotomist was located and that my results would be available by the end of the day. "I may get the results before they're posted on the portal," Shannon said. "If so, I'll call you when I get them. I know you must be anxious to hear."

That, my friends, was an accurate statement. At that point I was wishing I'd brought a Klonopin with me to keep my anxiety at bay.

I asked what Shannon wanted to see on the PSA test.

"At Sloan Kettering, we look for a PSA of less than 0.05, which is essentially undetectable."

"Zero point oh-five," I repeated back to her.

"*Less than* 0.05," Shannon corrected me. "We need to see that less than symbol or it's not really undetectable."

So that was the magic number—the pole I had to limbo under to continue my life with some degree of optimism. My brain latched on to it like Frodo clutching his magic ring.

Eventually, I was released to go home. My return to Saratoga that afternoon was uneventful. During the three-hour drive, I texted Barbara for updates on the symposium and shared my news about the "wisp." Her reports on the symposium were exultant: The keynote address was standing room only and overall attendance was better than their most hopeful projections. Buoyed by her good fortune, I disclosed that I'd given blood for my six-week PSA but didn't have results yet. Not wanting to distract her from the success of her event, I tried to sound upbeat. She, in turn, sent encouraging messages whenever she had a break between presentations. As the town car made its way to Saratoga, I distracted myself by making small-talk with my driver. However, I quickly learned that his politics were anathema to mine, so I switched to reading the news on my iPhone. At around 3 PM we pulled up outside my home.

The house was empty, of course. Late-afternoon sunshine slanted through the windows in the family room where our big siamese cat, Winston, was asleep on the sofa. Our other cat, a tiny Abyssinian named Gita, had curled up in a warm square of light by the French doors. Neither took notice of me when I opened the front door and set the mail on the dining room table. In the kitchen I saw signs of the activity that must have preceded Barbara's departure for the symposium: coffee mugs and cereal bowls in the sink, Merle's copy of the keynote speaker's book on the kitchen counter. Unsettled and anxious, I grabbed my laptop and a glass of ice water, headed into the family room, and turned on the TV. Taking a deep breath, I logged in to the MSK portal and went right to the Lab Results section.

Nothing had been posted.

As was the case when Shannon appeared not to have my pathology results a few weeks earlier, I felt a wave of relief not to find anything. The fact is, ever since I gave blood that morning at Sloan Kettering, I'd had a nagging feeling my results would be bad. It wasn't entirely irrational, either: With the exception of my post-surgical pathology report, every PSA test, biopsy report, and MRI had yielded progressively worse news. There had been a menacing trajectory to this cancer, and on some level I acknowledged that one good report hadn't changed that reality.

Intent on distracting myself from these ruminations, I browsed the on-demand movies on our cable TV and came across *Wonder*, starring Owen Wilson and Julia Roberts. It sounded appropriately innocuous, so I watched the trailer. From what I could tell, it was a formulaic tear-jerker about a little boy with a facial disfigurement and his experience of entering the public school system after years of sheltered homeschooling. It looked like it ended happily, which was absolutely essential for today's viewing, so I ponied up the rental fee of $5.95 and settled in with my laptop nearby.

Every 15 minutes or so, I'd pause the movie and log back into the MSK portal, each time finding no results posted. The movie, meanwhile, was proving an excellent choice, with all the usual Hollywood mechanisms for evoking a sigh of sympathy or a gasp of indignation. The precocious little boy, with a face disfigured just enough to render him at once startling and adorable, teaches those around him the meaning of dignity and perseverance. His first few weeks at school see him bullied and mocked by mean kids, and heartbreakingly betrayed by his new best friend. His older sister, feeling overshadowed by the boy's disability, struggles in her own right to overcome a failed friendship on the one hand and be open to romance on the other.

For someone looking to fire up all the positive emotions, this movie had it all.

Around 4:10, as the movie was winding down, I logged into the portal again, went into Lab Results and, before I even registered what I was looking at, saw an entry dated 3/23/18.

"Prostate Specific AntiGEN (PSA) <0.05ng/ml"

The notation was so brief I took it for a caption detailing the target PSA level. No test results yet, just a reiteration of the critical benchmark.

Then I read it again.

Below the notation, a disclaimer read, "Results cannot be interpreted as evidence of the presence or absence of malignant disease. Assay info: IEMA,Tosoh AIA."

It said *results*.

I sat up and leaned into the computer, scrutinizing the entry over and over again. My eyes returned obsessively to the "less than" sign, as if it might creep off the screen when I wasn't looking. Finally satisfied my imagination wasn't playing tricks on me, I looked over at Winston asleep on the couch. "Well, goddamn," I said to him. "*Goddamn.*"

The sun had dipped behind the leafless maple trees in the empty lot to our west, and the light spilling in the windows was now dappled and pale. The weather that day had been neither warm nor cold—it was one of those uniquely northeastern days when the snow lingering in the backyard denoted winter, but the gemlike quality of the sunlight and the scent in the air promised spring. For a moment, I studied the shards of pale, white light on our hardwood floor, then, rousing myself as if from a pleasant daydream, took up my phone and thumb-typed a note to Barbara. "Good news on PSA!" I texted. Then I sent the same note to Mattie.

Moments later, I received an almost audible "OMG" from Barbara. Barbara's use of text shortcuts was uncharacteristic, which indicated she was probably tied up in conversations with symposium attendees. I could imagine her sneaking peeks at her phone throughout the afternoon, torn between feeling triumphant over her event and anxious about my imminent test results. Again, I found myself regretting the encroachment of my cancer on her happiness. *At least*, I thought, *the news was good and could only add to her buoyancy.*

A moment later, Mattie texted back with at least five heart-eyed smiley faces and, characteristically, a quick succession of questions about the test results, how I was feeling, and when she would see me next. As fast as I could type an answer, my phone pinged with another question, and another. Finally, she punctuated our exchange with, "I am sooooo happy!" I could feel her relief in that long series of "o's." Relief may have been everyone's prevailing emotion at that point. Genuine happiness took longer to seep in.

Barbara then surprised me by texting that Daniel Quinn, my retired doctor whose recommendation to get a PSA test probably saved my life, was attending her symposium and sent his best. It seemed wonderfully appropriate that Dr. Quinn re-entered the picture that day, five months after the whole thing started. I knew that he, too, had prostate cancer, so I made a mental note to call him soon to catch up.

Next, I sent a short text to my siblings and sat there enjoying the chime of my phone as responses of "YAY!!!" and "AMAZING!!!" came through.

My good news shared with loved ones and warm waves of relief flooding over me like a morphine shot, I settled into my chair to finish the movie. The little boy gets his best friend back and wins over his enemies by standing up against tough kids from a competing school. His sister finds love and joins the drama club, giving a bravura performance in the school play. The emotional crescendo is a year-end awards ceremony where the school principal announces that the recipient of the character award, given for showing true courage in the face of daunting circumstances, is the little boy.

Owen Wilson grins triumphantly. Julia Roberts puts her hands to her cheeks and weeps with joy. Every loose end is tied up neatly.

My reaction, I believe, started when the principal gave his speech; but it really kicked in when the crowd burst into applause and the boy realized he'd won the award.

I sobbed.

Now, this wasn't the usual moist eye after a happy ending. It was something entirely new and wholly unexpected: a spasm in my chest and shoulders, and the distinct sensation of having a stopper pulled out of a cavity deep inside my body. Four months of emotion seemed to pour out of me like the swallows at San Juan Capistrano. I was a hot mess, sitting there with stinging cheeks and a runny nose, smiling and weeping at the little kid as he accepted his courage award.

Shocked by this emotional outpouring, I recalled Harry Sanborn in *Something's Gotta Give*, my go-to movie for twenty-first-century philosophical reference points. After surviving a heart attack, Harry can't figure out why he cries for no apparent reason. He thanks his doctor and he cries. He has sex with Erica and he cries. It's as if his emotions became an Aeolian harp, sounding off with the merest hint of a breeze. In just thirty seconds, I concluded, I had become a movie cliché. As surprised as I was by this sudden emotionality, I didn't mind it. In fact, I welcomed the unburdening, not much caring whether I wept because the movie was uplifting or my wife had a great day or my test results came out right. Or whatever.

When my body decided I was done with my impromptu catharsis, I wiped my face, blew my nose, and put away my laptop, taking a last look at the test score just to be sure. Then my phone rang, the caller ID indicating it was Touijer's office.

"Mr. Hill? It's Shannon from Dr. Touijer's office. I wanted to let you know that your PSA results are back." Before I could tell her I'd seen the portal, she continued. "It's really good news. It came back as undetectable."

"Oh, man, that's fantastic, Shannon."

"I know it's getting a little late, but I wanted to call right away when I saw. I hope that makes your weekend a little brighter."

"That's for sure. Thank you so much, Shannon. And please

thank Dr. Touijer. You all have been amazing. I'll see you next week?"

As far as I was concerned, I didn't mind receiving the PSA results over and over again—like how I re-read the sports page when the Broncos beat the Packers to win their first Super Bowl. I couldn't get enough.

In the kitchen I refilled my glass of ice water and headed for the bathroom to empty my catheter bag. The Foley and I would be together for another five days, at the end of which the catheter would be uneventfully—and permanently—removed. I had months more of Kegel exercises and discreet absorbent "shields" still ahead. And, of course, thanks to my friends at the Sexual Health Clinic, I could look forward to three penile injections every week to remind me that healing was a marathon, not a sprint. In a week or so, I could resume normal exercise and socializing without a secret pouch strapped to my left leg. In another six months, I'd repeat the PSA test—and then again and again for the rest of my life. For now, though, I had a calmness of spirit so unfamiliar that I scarcely recognized it. I looked forward to later that evening when Barbara, Merle, and Sue would get home and we could sit in the family room and talk indulgently about the symposium, the serendipity of Dr. Quinn attending, the brilliance and generosity of the keynote speaker, our good luck with the weather—anything other than catheters, prostate cancer, or the depredations of aging. Today, at least, the cosmic joker's attention was turned elsewhere and the threat of irony could be momentarily disregarded. I knew, as Barbara did, that misfortune was never far away and old age lay ahead like a heavy fog on the road. But for now, screw it. It felt good just to sweep the spiders of fear from my mind.

Around 6:30 I heard the tires of Barbara's car crunching on the gravel in our driveway and went to unlock the side door. In the glow of the porch light, I could see Barbara and Merle walking up the stone path, talking energetically. Sue walked a step behind them, looking down and listening intently. All three were buzzing with excitement over the symposium's success. In that moment, as I watched them mount the stairs to the door, I regained some part of me that had been lost for months.

EPILOGUE

WHEN I WAS A KID in Denver, my best friend John and I set up a skateboard slalom course on the sidewalk along 17th Avenue, around the corner from my house. Having decided we were ready for something more challenging than rolling around our neighborhood streets, we collected a bunch of Campbell's soup cans, washed them out, peeled off the labels, and spray-painted them bright red. One hot July afternoon, John and I packed the cans into a grocery bag and headed down Monaco Parkway toward 17th Avenue to set up the course. As I arranged the cans on the long stretch of concrete, John stepped back to assess the intervals and see whether they looked about right for our skill level. We eventually settled on a course that ran about half the length of the block and consisted of sixteen gates. We thought it looked pretty easy.

John volunteered to take the first run and readied himself at the starting line. Holding a stopwatch I had borrowed from my brother David, who ran track in high school, I took my position at the other end of the course and gave John the ready, set, go.

Neither one of us was a highly skilled skateboarder. We didn't have access to the impressive skateboard parks you see these days, so mostly we skated in the bank parking lot and on a newly paved stretch of Krameria Street, a few blocks from my house. John's first run was actually pretty good. He navigated most of the gates successfully, only missing a couple toward the end, and cruised through the finish line, sweaty and grinning. Convinced I could hit all the gates on my first run, I grabbed my skateboard—a double-kick-tail, aluminum Banzai with red polyurethane wheels—and positioned myself at the starting line. John took his place at the end of the course with the stopwatch.

I put my board down and placed my right foot squarely in its center, flexing my sneakered toes against strips of textured tape on the aluminum deck.

"Ready . . . set . . . GO!"

With great sweeps of my left foot, I took off like a missile, anticipating the first turn with the concentration of an Olympic skier. I cleared the initial gates reasonably well, but each time I swerved around a can, my turns became wider, causing me to lose speed. Two thirds into the course, I decided slalom was a lot harder than it looked—and John was better than I gave him credit for. Just as that thought struck me, my wheel hit a pebble on the sidewalk and all hell broke loose. There was a sharp grating sound of stone on concrete as my front wheel seized up. In an instant, my board flipped out from under me and sailed into the grass by the sidewalk. Meanwhile, I catapulted down the sidewalk, wiping out two cans and coming to rest 10 feet past my upended Banzai, its red wheels still spinning. A sharp pain on my right elbow revealed a nasty abrasion oozing blood. *Somewhere along that sidewalk,* I thought, *I had left a significant patch of skin.*

My cheeks burning with frustration, I mumbled some teenager's curse words, gathered myself up, and retrieved my skateboard. Thinking I would take another run at the course, I started to search for the offending pebble but quickly realized my arm hurt too much to continue. So, five minutes after laying them out, we gathered up our soup cans and returned them to the grocery bag, pledging to sweep the sidewalk next time. John must have felt pretty good about his only run and treated me with guarded magnanimity, asking if he should carry my skateboard and urging me to clean the gravel out of my wound. On the way back to the house, I regained my composure and even managed to joke about being momentarily airborne before I crashed. I don't think we ever tried a slalom course again.

Every now and then, when I'm washing my arms after an ambitious day in the garden, I'll rediscover the scar from my skateboarding accident. My collision with the sidewalk those many years ago removed about a square inch of skin, and the oozy wound took weeks to form a thick scab and eventually heal over. I was left with an odd patch of bumpy ostrich skin. When my arm is bent, I can see the scar quite clearly; when my arm is extended, the glossy tissue crinkles up and disappears. Every time I chance upon this badge of skateboarding impetuosity, my mind races back to that hot afternoon, the massive elm trees that lined 17th Avenue, the buzz of insects in the July air, the red soup cans, and curly-haired John readying his skateboard for the first run.

I have an array of other scars, of course, though few evoke such vivid memories. I also have marks that are complete mysteries, like the odd divot on my forehead, the origin of which eludes me to this day, or the three-quarter-inch furrow on top of my right hand. But mostly I remember the stories of my scars, life's capricious inscriptions on the palimpsest that is my body. There is the place I had a granuloma removed from my left cheek when I was in college. My father, I later learned, was terrified the bump might be cancerous and suffered through two anguished days before learning it was a harmless blob of tissue that had formed around some debris in a pore. On my right palm, there is a diagonal slash where, as a 16-year-old stumbling around in my dark bedroom, I fell on a terrarium, shattering the glass as I broke my fall. I had turned on the light in a panic and seen a triangular shard of glass stuck in my flesh, blood pooling in my hand like water from a spring. I have more recent scars on each of my shins from jumping on—and missing—tall metal platforms used in fitness sessions at the Y. My first miss resulted in a painful contusion on the left shin. A year later, I foolishly attempted jumping with one leg after seeing a guy in his 20s do the same thing. A guy in his 50s should have probably known better. I ended up with a two-inch gash in my right shin that required stitches at the urgent care center. Those memories involve equal measures of pain and embarrassment.

Now, of course, I have five new marks on my abdomen from the prostatectomy. The three smaller scars, all of them neat, horizontal lines, have now faded to a light pink. Where Touijer made his biggest incision—a vertical cut running a fraction of an inch to the left of my navel—the color is still vivid purple, though largely hidden beneath a swirl of stomach hair. Below that scar is a small fifth incision, also vertical, that was the first to heal. When I carry a little extra weight in my midsection, the scars become dimples, reminding me to pass on the duck-fat french fries at The Brook Tavern. Unlike other scars that are the products of life's little accidents, these new marks are orderly—manmade and intentional—bespeaking their origin in a very different set of circumstances. Consequently, when, after a shower, I gaze at my newly inscribed midsection, my mind doesn't teem with nostalgic reveries the way it does with my skateboarding scar. The new marks don't conjure memories of my diagnosis or the night after surgery when I needed Barbara's help getting into bed. Instead, I tend to gaze at myself in an act of reassessment, as if the scars are serial numbers on the new body I've been assigned by the divine manufacturer. Where I came to regard other marks on my body as corporeal footnotes to a life story I understood and largely controlled, these new entries changed the narrative entirely. In fact, since their appearance, I almost don't recognize the story at all.

Assessing how I came to this point of relative bemusement, I can't blame the cancer entirely. As I explained earlier, the midpoint of my life had already presented strange new challenges that forced me to re-examine my identity, my life's ambition, and even my understanding of the past. When the cancer diagnosis arrived just before Christmas of 2017, it became another layer on the heap of existential considerations I already pondered daily. In that sense, I suppose, prostate cancer became a kind of emblem for midlife—at least for mine. If I was already feeling attenuated as a result of being 56, cancer made me feel more so. If I was already preoccupied with mortality, cancer filled me with vivid new urgency. Nearly every concern that my illness presented or intensified was already on my mind; and my initiation into the mystery cult of cancer gave me a comprehensive paradigm in which to function and into which I organized my anxieties.

Foremost among these newly vivified anxieties was the issue of masculinity and what it looks like, feels like, in middle age and, in particular, after prostate cancer treatment. I mentioned earlier that, during my illness, Mattie shared with me various readings from her sociology courses at Barnard. She knew I had become interested in race and gender issues, so she occasionally passed along relevant articles from her syllabus. In particular, I was interested in sociological perspectives on gender construction and the roles society expects men and women to "perform" in sustaining millennia-old patterns of human interchange. Until reading more deeply in this subject, I had never viewed my masculine self as a *role* I played or as something distinguishable from my more elemental self; nor did I consider the possibility that much of my professional, physical, or even romantic ambition in life had been fueled by American cultural expectations. My readings on gender roles presented an entirely new way of viewing how I had conducted my life for over five decades—why I made certain decisions and why I sometimes felt a schism between the public-facing man I had become, and who I had hoped to be. This lens gave me sharp new perspective on the seismic transformation I underwent with the near-simultaneous occurrences of leaving business and being treated for prostate cancer, and how that change of roles affected my sense of prestige, self-confidence, and overall potency—in the figurative sense—as a man.

When I exited my career in marketing, I left more than a job. I stepped away from an entire performance—in the sociological sense—of myself as traditional success: I was a business owner who had made some decent money by building and selling a thriving enterprise. I was the husband of a beautiful, accomplished scholar whose success reflected on me as her choice of spouse. I was the father of a bright, confident young woman who attended college at an elite institution and whose sensibility and achievements validated my decisions as a parent and a husband. I loved my family, served for over a decade on the board of a non-profit organization, rode horses, shot sporting clays, exercised consistently, and had 1.5 cocktails at the end of most days. Over the course of six months, all those familiar bricks in the foundation of my masculine identity were rearranged, modified, or removed entirely. The result was uncertainty in virtually every part of my life. I came to question whether I would live past 60. I wondered whether I would regain my previous sexual health, if my private agony left me looking weak in Barbara's eyes, or if Mattie could forget seeing me frozen in agony on the bed amidst my folded clothes and suitcase. From a career perspective, I debated whether I should pursue my writing full-time or return to the type-A world of agency leadership. The common theme in these questions was masculinity and how it looks for someone whose career, outlook, and body had all been altered. For my own sanity, I needed to redefine masculinity to include the subtler attainments of aging: sagacity, patience, tenderness, compassion. As well, I think, I wanted affirmation that my culture values those qualities as highly as ambition, earning-power, and sexual aggression—the more customary manifestations of the male gender role. We'll see about that.

As vexing as the questions about masculinity were, midlife presented an even murkier outlook. I'd like to say that when I received my upbeat pathology report, followed by my six-week PSA results, the fog cleared from my perspective and I had a new sense of how to proceed with life. But that's not how it worked out. If cancer became the emblem for my midlife preoccupations, the apparent resolution of the cancer problem eliminated only the most immediate and threatening challenges. Life, as they say, goes on and, though I have gained an extraordinary new viewpoint as a result of my experience, the landscape of my future life remains nearly as shrouded in mist as when the journey began. The difference is that I'm not as worried about stumbling off a cliff as I figure out where the trail is. The question of where the trail lies, and where it leads, is as common to middle age as belly fat. Middle age marks that point in life when we begin to hear the ticking of the mortality clock as loudly as the drum of a woodpecker banging on our clapboards. And with that ticking comes a mild sense of panic that we haven't accomplished all we had hoped before we shuffle off this mortal coil—whether that means climbing Kilimanjaro, writing a novel, running a marathon, or whatever. So the introspective among us take that proverbial long, hard look at ourselves and make what we believe are the necessary course corrections. The objective in doing so, I suppose, is to avoid the classic deathbed regret—that one's life wasn't lived to its fullest.

My father, who, by any measure I can imagine, lived an extraordinarily full life, surprised me on this subject. It was April of 2014, a few weeks before he died from pancreatic cancer, and I was in Denver to spend some time with him and my siblings. Though my father was in a great deal of pain, he was still very much himself, engaging us in long conversations about my mother, his memories of the war, his ministry, and his cancer research. One evening he asked for help getting to bed, which I readily provided. When he finished his ablutions, I helped him take off his robe and ease under the covers. His cancer caused terrific pain in his lower back and abdomen, so getting comfortable was maddeningly elusive. As he settled in, frustrated by his frailty and grimacing from the pain, he put his hand on my arm in the darkness of his bedroom.

"Son," he said with an uncharacteristically defeated tone, "make sure you live your life before the hard times come."

So much about that statement struck me. Though I knew he had regrets about his life and all that befell him, it never occurred to me that someone with so many extraordinary accomplishments might go to his death feeling he hadn't lived "fully." Certainly, those of us who knew him couldn't imagine how he could have packed more into his life. Yet his accomplishments were, to a certain degree, achieved in defiance of his trials—like St. Augustine's *caritas*, a virtue borne, ironically, of misfortune. It's impossible to say how his life would have unfolded had he not lost a young wife and found himself alone and overwhelmed with five children, a mountain of medical debt, and a demanding new job. It never occurred to me, until his expression of regret, that he might have chosen a very different course for himself had life not thrown an arsenal of problems at him. His use of the term "hard times" also surprised me. Arguably, he had seen more "hard times" in his life than anyone I knew, and at an early age, too. In fact, he was defined by those grim experiences and how he—and his family—survived them. I'm certain, though, that he was referring to the last years of his life as the hardest, when, after my stepmother Nancy died of lupus, he found himself alone again and, eventually, came face to face with his old nemesis.

I often think back to my father's admonition, trying to parse what exactly he meant and how he viewed his life. If the hard times were the last few years of his life, I surmised, then all the misfortune that befell him at the midpoint of his life had somehow been revised, or become subsumed into a more positive assessment of the full arc of his existence. While extraordinary difficulties assaulted him, he continued to *live* in the very active sense of the verb. As he persisted, like an icebreaker shearing through a frozen sea, his misfortunes eventually gave way to a prevailing and tenacious sense of hope that the next day, month, or year could bring with it opportunity, however small, for happiness. The hard times came at the very end of his life, when—unless you drop dead from an aneurysm on the golf course or pass quietly in your sleep—the fact of mortality ordains we all face our greatest tribulations.

My Dad loved the poetry of Robinson Jeffers, particularly "The Deer Lay Down Their Bones." In the poem, the narrator reflects on the loss of his wife and the advance of old age, at last concluding, in defiance of his own suffering, "who drinks the wine / Should take the dregs; even in the bitter lees and sediment / New discovery may lie." My father referred to that poem more than once, so I inferred that it represented his own views on aging to some degree: No matter how discouraging life could be, no matter the losses one has suffered, on any given day there might still be something worth experiencing. Another phrase he used expressed that hopefulness from a more humorous perspective: When I complained that "life really sucks sometimes," he would respond, "It beats the alternative." That was the outlook of a man who had seen the worst that life could throw at a person and still kept looking for a break in the clouds.

I try to let that perspective guide me, particularly when, shaving in the morning, my eye falls upon my surgical scars and

I slip into the inevitable accounting of my own life. No doubt, middle age brings its indignities and depredations; and the path forward from this midpoint is through more perilous terrain than the path behind me. There's no getting around that reality. But there is also a fulsome quality to middle age. Maybe it's the "still sad music of humanity" Wordsworth refers to in "Lines Composed a Few Miles Above Tintern Abbey." When I read the poem cynically, I interpret that music as a dirge, but I don't think that's fair. What Wordsworth found, I think, was consolation for getting older—the "abundant recompense" he speaks of. He doesn't deny the profound sense of loss that comes with aging, and neither did my father. Growing old is tough, it's scary, and it comes with, seemingly, loss after loss.

For his consolation, Wordsworth turned to the power and majesty of nature and a divine power that "rolls through all things." I'm not at all religious, so when I look at nature, I see the same beauty the poet did, and I believe I derive a similar sense of serenity from sunsets and mountain vistas. But where Wordsworth saw godhead, I see a kind of roiling substratum of possibility—Aristotle's *potentia*—that imbues even the crappiest day with the chance that something good could still happen. Sure, I could wake up to another shit-storm like my cancer diagnosis or the day anxiety moved in as my emotional roommate. That's always a possibility. But so, too, is the chance that Barbara's cosmic joker will throw a little love my way and make something good, maybe even extraordinary, happen. Don't misunderstand me: That sense of possibility doesn't put some kind of Danny Kaye bounce in my step—I'll always tend toward the saturnine in my outlook—but it does console me.

As for prostate cancer, I'm still doing my Kegel exercises and wearing a thin absorbent pad in my boxer briefs to guard against an accidental drop when I laugh at a singing dog video. The constellation of scars on my abdomen is less noticeable by the day. My recovery is very much a work in progress and I'm okay with that because I do see progress. In three months, I'll have my six-month PSA test to see if my number is still the magic <0.05; and that promises to be a trying day. At those PSA tests, I meet with my remarkable surgeon Karim Touijer, and when I do, I'm reminded how fortunate I was to have found him and Memorial Sloan Kettering. Barbara once remarked that Dr. Touijer, his nurse practitioner Shannon, and their entire team made my treatment experience so much more tolerable than it might have otherwise been. For all my joking about his good looks and fighter-pilot confidence, I can't imagine finding a surgeon with a more dazzling combination of skill, decency, and compassion. I wish every prostate cancer patient could find the same level of care and kindness that I received.

In between those trips to Dr. Touijer, I continue with my injection therapy. Three times a week I retreat to my bedroom and gather my injection apparatus: one syringe, a bottle of the magic potion called Bimix, sterile alcohol wipes, and the Moleskine ledger in which I record the results of each shot, using MSK's one-to-ten scale. When I began the therapy, I agreed to participate in a study being conducted by the Sexual Health Clinic. Doing so involves speaking with a social worker named Diana, at first weekly and then monthly, about my progress, my emotional state, and my compliance with the program. I've been a good participant, I think, and my near-religious devotion to sticking a needle in my junk three times a week seems to stymie her. Each time we talk, I feel I should give Diana more to ask about. After all, I'm on a tiny 5-unit dose, achieve eight- and nine-point erections without fail, and seldom miss an injection. Perhaps at some point, I'll miss a week to give us something to dig into. It's not all smooth sailing, though. Diana encourages me, in her classic Long Island accent, to trot out these impressive woodies for real-world use—an undertaking that has, for obvious reasons, felt fraught with complexity, both emotional and practical. "Okay, honey, I just dropped the syringe in the sharps container and I'm ready for action" just doesn't sound like the start of a romantic interlude. I've got a lot of confidence to recover in that area. I'm relieved to say, however, that my rehab has advanced to the point where I'm nearly good to go without a shot. So, in my most optimistic moods, I view the injections as a way to keep things improving. Who knows, maybe I'll wind up better off than I was before—the way my friend Terry did with his stallion-stream urinations. I doubt it, though—his story was a rarity in all the prostate cancer narratives I read. For me, it's better and more realistic to hope for a return to my previous functionality. Though the shots won't last forever (thank God), I can say there is some satisfaction in experiencing the kind of tentpole most men don't see after 30.

As encouraging as the teenager-quality stiffies are, however, it's no picnic giving myself shots. You never really get used to sticking a needle in your private parts. Having been instructed to alternate sides each day, I dread when I must clumsily administer the injection left-handed. If I hit a vein, there is bleeding. If I use too much alcohol, I get a stinger. After giving myself a shot, the objective is to maintain an erection of six or better for fifteen to thirty minutes. Afterwards, I emerge sheepishly from the bedroom, still feeling a lingering tumescence that will require another hour to disappear completely. Barbara is unfazed by this ritual, having grown accustomed, perhaps more than I, to the strange rhythms of recovery from prostate cancer. If she is reading in her study, she might look up as I pass by on the way to the bathroom. "How'd it go?" she'll ask.

"Got an eight today." And with that casual exchange, we return to living life between the margins of cancer.

All things considered, I think of myself as a very, very lucky man. Had Dr. Quinn not urged me to get a PSA test, I would probably still have an undetected malignancy on the left side of my prostate, perhaps even metastases to my bones or organs. Having gotten the "all clear" on my digital rectal exam back in the fall of 2017, I'd still be cruising through life, oblivious to the looming threat—just like that car in the Grant Wood painting.

So, no, my experience of prostate cancer was wholly unlike what I read in the books or blogs. It was more complicated, more nuanced, more painful, more emotionally challenging than I ever expected. It was sadder, funnier, stranger, more disappointing, and more encouraging than I could have imagined. Yet here I am, about six months since my diagnosis, and I find myself at times slipping into some of the same euphemisms about prostate cancer I've come to despise. I'll be sitting at dinner with friends who ask how I'm doing and the platitudes kick in like a bad habit: a valiant smile and a dismissive wave of the hand when speaking vaguely of "side effects," or the self-effacing and inauthentic relief that it wasn't "something more serious." Maybe I reserve all my candor for the pages of this book. After all, telling someone about your terrifying Gleason score, bladder leak, catheterizations, penile injections, or leaky plumbing doesn't make for great conversation over artisanal pizza and Chianti. As I said, it's difficult for men to talk candidly about health concerns at all, much less the surprises that come with this disease. After some initial alarm and confusion about how real, scary, and complicated prostate cancer is, it's natural for us just to focus on getting better and let the next guy figure it out for himself. I guess the alarm I felt after *my* first few surprises sustained itself long enough for me to start writing this book.

Since I began writing, I've heard many stories about men who have been diagnosed with prostate cancer. It's like the Baader-Meinhof phenomenon when, after you decide to buy a Toyota SUV, seemingly every other car you see on the road is a Highlander. I just never paid attention to how prevalent prostate cancer is. I hear men speak, often with uncharacteristic resignation, about all they didn't know, their struggles to get past lingering urinary or potency problems, the strain on their families and relationships, the impact on their self-esteem. That's the stuff that breaks my heart and reminds me that, in the spirit of the Dalai Lama and his belief in our interconnectedness, we men need to pass the word. Let the next guy know that the "good cancer" can be really bad; that you're probably going to feel banged up and emasculated at times; that you'll wonder on which examination room floor you left your dignity like a rumpled pile of clothes.

Mostly I just want to let other men know I went through the same thing and, for now at least, came out in one piece.

TAKEAWAYS FOR MEN OVER 50

AS I MENTIONED in my introduction, I want *Midpoint* to be the book I looked for but couldn't find when I was diagnosed with prostate cancer. And, while the book touches on all the points I make below, I wanted to put them in one place for reference. This advice is based only on my experience, of course. You're a different person with a different set of circumstances, so your main partner in all health discussions is your physician, with whom you should have a comfortable, candid, and open relationship. If you don't have that, switch doctors.

OVER-50 MEN'S HEALTH IN GENERAL:

1.   **OWN YOUR HEALTH CARE.** Know the recommended screenings for your age and request them from your doctor. Acquaint yourself with the target ranges for every screening and be engaged when the results come back. Take notes. Ask questions.

2.   **GET A PHYSICAL EVERY 12 MONTHS.** And make sure prostate health is on the agenda every visit.

3.   **HAVE YOUR PSA TESTED EVERY YEAR.** Remember that your results may need to be confirmed or corrected by a follow-up screening.

If you're over 70, your doctor may recommend against PSA testing, a position that has real merit. Have the conversation either way, and select a strategy together.

4. DON'T FREAK OUT IF YOUR RESULTS COME BACK HIGH. Remember that PSA isn't unique to prostate cancer. It can be caused by several other conditions such as normal aging, benign prostatic hyperplasia, prostatitis, or a urinary tract infection.

IF YOUR PSA IS CONFIRMED AS ABNORMALLY HIGH:

1. BRING A SPOUSE, PARTNER, OR OTHER LOVED ONE TO *ALL* MAJOR APPOINTMENTS. They're critical both for moral support and as a second set of ears when you may be distracted.

2. LOOK INTO GETTING AN MRI BEFORE A BIOPSY. Your insurance plan may not cover an MRI, but don't give up. If your request is denied by your plan, appeal. If you can afford it, pay out of pocket. An MRI may show that no biopsy is required. It will also help get a more accurate needle biopsy, if one is recommended.

3. IF YOU PROCEED TO BIOPSY, ASK FOR MILD SEDATION. Biopsies can be pretty uncomfortable. Also, prepare yourself to see blood in your stools and semen after the procedure.

IF YOU ARE DIAGNOSED WITH PROSTATE CANCER:

1. STAY CALM AND DO YOUR HOMEWORK. Read as much good, reputable information as you can find about treatment options, and come to the process educated and willing to learn more.

2. CONTINUE BRINGING THAT LOVED ONE WITH YOU TO APPOINTMENTS. Take notes. Ask questions. Expect excellence and compassion from every person you deal with. You have that right.

3. CHOOSE A TREATMENT PLAN FOR *YOUR* CANCER. Once you're diagnosed, you may get advice from lots of other men, which is helpful. But your cancer is unique and requires a plan designed around your special profile as a patient.

4.   WHEN SELECTING A SURGEON OR RADIATION ONCOLOGIST, BE PICKY AS HELL. There is absolutely no reason to compromise—and every reason to persevere. Look for someone who is expert in your chosen treatment with a *verifiable* record of success.

5.   BE YOUR OWN ADVOCATE. Ask for copies of all test results, instructions, recommendations, etc. Don't be passive. Doctors aren't perfect, and they may not automatically communicate everything you'd want.

6.   BE A MODEL PATIENT. Follow your doctor's recommendations for preparation and recovery. It's your *body*, not a math test in high school, so don't take shortcuts. The only person who suffers when you get lazy is you.

7.   BE KIND TO YOURSELF. Wherever your cancer takes you, remember that human beings do best when surrounded by loved ones and compassionate caregivers. Confide in someone you trust. Allow yourself time to process what you're going through. It's a lot to take in, and the presence and support of others is absolutely irreplaceable.

If you have prostate cancer, you're not alone: There are 2.9 million men living with the disease today and another 165,000 will be diagnosed this year. For me, at least, it helped to remember that it's a common disease for men and the vast majority of men have excellent outcomes.

ACKNOWLEDGMENTS

ANYONE WHO HAS BEEN TREATED for cancer has a lot of thank you's to say. Ironically, I don't know the names of many people who helped me through this strange odyssey. There are dozens of individuals at Memorial Sloan Kettering and other health care facilities who answered phones, ushered me into examination rooms, took blood, administered MRIs, carried me down stairs to an ambulance, scheduled appointments, and generally made the whole experience tolerable. The American healthcare system, however complex and maddening at times, employs some amazingly dedicated people. I am particularly appreciative for the talented Dr. Karim Touijer and his entire staff at MSK. I have seldom encountered a kinder or more capable group of people in a more unexpected setting. Likewise, I must acknowledge the team at MSK's Sexual Health Clinic. Through their compassion and patience, they managed to make the strangest aspect of this whole process seem, well, perfectly fine. I will always be profoundly grateful to my former primary care physician, referred to in this book as Dr. Daniel Quinn, for two decades of excellent care and, most notably, for urging me to get that fateful PSA test. Of course my siblings, David, Kristin, Cydney, and Geoffrey, have all been a source of strength as I fretted over various procedures and test results. Geoff mysteriously managed to know when all my major screenings were scheduled, and called or texted to give me moral support. Thanks, as well, to Terry Julius and Frank Cristiano for their insight on prostate cancer treatment, and for sharing their stories with me.

Sadly, the people who get bruised up the most in an experience like mine are one's immediate family. My daughter Madeleine saw more scary stuff than any father would wish, but her encouragement always managed to brighten my outlook. As for my wife Barbara, she was nothing less than my lodestar, providing counsel, love, and tenacious hopefulness—even when I got gloomy or short-tempered. Her remarkable support extended beyond my cancer treatment: Over the course of twelve months, she read every word in this book multiple times, providing her marvelous English professor's insight into my often undisciplined prose. If prostate cancer taught me anything, it's how lucky I am to have married well.

CPSIA information can be obtained
at www.ICGtesting.com
Printed in the USA
LVHW050457261119
638500LV00006B/358/P